PRAISE

Incurable Optimist

"This book is an inspiration. Read it to find your own bravery and to salute the bravery of Jennifer Cramer-Miller."

—DELIA EPHRON, author of *Left on Tenth:
A Second Chance at Life*

"A raw, heartfelt, and transformational read for anyone needing levity in the face of adversity. I love how Jennifer's humor-laced resilience beautifully encourages the reader to always make room for joy and hope!"

—JULIE BURTON, author of *The Self-Care Solution: A Modern
Mother's Must-Have Guide to Health and Well-Being*
and owner of ModernWell

"This book! Omg! The triumph of this journey! . . . a JOYOUS story . . ."

—LINDA SIVERTSEN, author, co-author, and ghostwriter of eleven
books including two NYT bestsellers, and host of the
Beautiful Writers Podcast

"Wonderful! I started crying so many times as I read . . . engaging, moving, funny."

—KATE HOPPER, author of *Ready for Air: A Journey through
Premature Motherhood* and *Use Your Words:
A Writing Guide for Mothers*

"If you ever want to read an inspirational book, and occasionally laugh out loud, I encourage you to read Jennifer Cramer-Miller's memoir. It is uplifting and gives new meaning to the word 'hope.'"

—HERTA FEELY, author of 2018 National Indie Excellence Award
and 2016 New Apple Award Winner *Saving Phoebe Murrow*

"In this deftly crafted memoir, Jennifer Cramer-Miller takes us on her volatile journey of navigating a chronic, life-threatening disease. Generously infused with humor and hard-won wisdom, *Incurable Optimist* reminds us that hope—and human connection—can help us overcome insurmountable odds. An insightful, inspiring, and joy-filled read."

—LAURA WHITFIELD, author of *Untethered: Faith, Failure, and Finding Solid Ground*

"Jennifer Cramer Miller's optimism is born of living with reality, with the operative word being *living*. Anyone dealing with disappointment, hopelessness, or fear will be inspired by Jennifer's infectious optimism."

—BETSY GRAZIANI FASBINDER, author of three books including *Filling Her Shoes: A Memoir of an Inherited Family*, and podcast host of the Morning Glory Project

"Beyond inspiring—a page turner that reveals the resilience of the human spirit surrounded by unconditional love and support. Great read."

—AMY S. PEELE, award-winning author of a medical murder mystery trilogy, *Cut, Match*, and *Hold*

"If you're looking for a wonderful, uplifting, and real look at what it's like to be living with illness, look no further. With a crystal-clear writing style, Jennifer Cramer Miller describes the fears and desperation after diagnosis while bravely holding onto resilience, joy, and hope."

—JULIE JO SEVERSON, author of *Oldest-Twin Cities: A Guide to Historic Treasures* and co-author of *Here in the Middle: Stories of Love, Loss, and Connection from the Ones Sandwiched in Between*

Incurable
Optimist

Incurable
Optimist

Living with Illness
and
Chronic Hope

Jennifer Cramer-Miller

SHE WRITES PRESS

Published 2023
Printed in the United States of America
Print ISBN: 978-1-64742-527-2
E-ISBN: 978-1-64742-528-9
Library of Congress Control Number: 2023906715

For information, address:
She Writes Press
1569 Solano Ave #546
Berkeley, CA 94707

Interior design by Stacey Aaronson

She Writes Press is a division of SparkPoint Studio, LLC.

Author's Note

This book recounts my journey with kidney failure. Although I've navigated a rocky road since the age of twenty-two, my socioeconomic status and skin color were not roadblocks along the way. Unfortunately, this is not the case for many of my fellow kidney patients.

Currently serving as the Minnesota Board Chair for the National Kidney Foundation, I know that Black individuals have a three to four times higher rate of kidney failure than whites. Hispanic and Latino individuals have a 1.3 times higher rate than whites. Native Americans, Asian Americans, and Pacific Islanders also face a higher risk of kidney disease. Yet there are disparities in access to care. That's why the National Kidney Foundation and kidney community are focused on improving health care equity and accessibility.

I'm excited about the innovations in the works to benefit kidney patients. Portable dialysis machines are ahead, and eventually, bioengineered kidneys could eliminate waiting lists and immunosuppressive medications. Hope is on the horizon. Both now and in the future, equal access is essential so that the best treatments benefit kidney health for all.

This is a work of nonfiction—a true story shared from my memory. We know memories are imperfect. Even so, I relied on mine (as well as notes and journals I'd kept along the way). The color of a shirt or the exact words spoken may not be exact (I didn't record and photograph everything, after all), but the essence is accurate. Plus, I have scrambled a few names and identifying details to protect the privacy of select individuals.

It is also worth noting that I am not a doctor, so nothing in this book about my health experiences should be considered medical advice or expertise. In addition, I speak for only myself and do not represent the views, positions, or endorsements of any organizations.

A final note of clarification: In 2017, the Minneapolis Park Board changed the name of Lake Calhoun (referenced in this book) to Bde Maka Ska, which restores the original Dakota name in honor of the Dakota people. When the events in this book took place, however, the name was Lake Calhoun, so I wrote this name for accuracy.

For Dirk and Liza

"If there's anything half so much fun as being alive,
I'd like to know what it is."

—FREDERICK BUECHNER

PART ONE

———

FAILING

"There is nothing certain, but the uncertain."

—Proverb

1.

Fallout

ONE MORNING AT THE TAIL END OF MY TWENTY-SECOND year, while downing coffee with my roommate, my face felt peculiar. Squishy. Leaning toward Lisa over the table in our apartment's tiny kitchen, I said, "Check this out. Don't my eyes look smaller?"

"Too much salt?" Lisa asked, before blowing steam from the top of her mug.

"Maybe." I pressed my fingers into the puffy skin that surrounded my upper and lower lashes.

It was Saturday, my energy lagged, and the warm cocoon of my duvet called. Eventually, I motivated myself to shower under a flow of hot water and throw on jeans and a chunky November-style sweater. Another glance in the mirror. Typically, I would blame a little puffiness on the regular suspects, PMS or MSG. But on this day, the skin around my eyes resembled spongy marshmallows.

I wondered if more coffee might help. It didn't. My brain felt as dull as the Seattle sky outside the apartment windows, where falling raindrops played percussion on glass. Lisa took off to hawk hosiery during her Nordstrom shift downtown. I stayed in. As the hours ticked by, my legs felt tight, and my inner voice vacillated between calm dismissal (it's nothing) and far-flung possibilities (bubonic plague?). I had no idea to what extent—but I was not okay.

Sprawled on the couch with the television on, I called my boyfriend, Nick, and vented about my dilemma.

"I'll come over tonight with some booze to flush you out," he offered, sounding lighthearted.

"Skip the booze. Just come over," I said, pressing my lips together. "There's no party potential tonight."

Six months earlier, Lisa and I had graduated from college. I met Nick in college too, but with more credits to complete, he still lived close to campus, thirty-five miles south of our apartment.

That night, after Lisa came home from work, Nick arrived with a bottle of wine. The three of us sank comfortably into the couch, but my mind was far from relaxed. Although I tried to silence my inner alarm, my eyes seemed worse, the skin around my ankles felt taut, and I had no fitting reference for these symptoms.

"Drink up." Nick handed me a glass filled to the brim.

"Jen, wine won't do it. You need a doctor," Lisa said firmly.

"I don't have one." During the past four years of college, the student health building was an easy walk across campus. But I hadn't needed a doctor since graduation, and as a recent resident of Seattle, I knew nothing of the city's medical clinics.

"Get one."

The next day, I dialed my parents and explained that I felt off. "Maybe I'm coming down with the flu?" I said in a measured voice. I didn't want to alarm them, but that didn't work. Although their Minnesota home was miles from Washington, they jumped into action.

Monday morning, Dad reported he'd gotten a referral to a Seattle internist from his doctor in Minneapolis. They set an appointment for the next day, Tuesday, at 11:00. I noted it on my calendar and dashed out the door so I wouldn't be late for work. I snagged the bus from our Capitol Hill apartment to my office in Pioneer Square, where I worked as a public relations intern.

Same routine as always. I raced into the building on Occidental Avenue, jogged through the lobby to catch the elevator, and stepped into the office on the sixth floor where everyone buzzed—twenty or so professional bees in a frenzy of creative production. After some quick nods to the bigwigs in a conference room on the perimeter of the open space, I sat at my designated intern cubicle. I resumed updating a CEO database and tried to ignore my swollen eyes, feet, and fingers.

I was excited about this choice internship at Cole & Weber, a subsidiary of a national PR firm, Ogilvy & Mather. When my boss, Stacy, selected me from two hundred applicants, I let out an involuntary squeal and shimmied a happy dance. With my foot in the door and my work in the mix, I planned to secure a future position. I wanted to put my newly earned business degree to work. So I intended to be the perfect intern.

That's why I reluctantly approached Stacy to tell her I had a doctor's appointment the next day and had to leave before my lunch break. She tried to scrutinize my face, but I lowered my head. Fine with me if she saw the same hard-to-tame, medium-length brunette hair and freckles splattered on my nose—but I didn't want her to stare at the swelling surrounding my brown eyes. "Everything okay?" she asked. She was three years older, and our relationship was strictly professional. But at this moment, she seemed more concerned about me than my performance.

I forced a perky tone. "Oh, I think so. Just need to be sure."

My daytime internship was for career advancement, but the pay wasn't much. So at night I sold costume jewelry and taffeta prom dresses at a department store. Late '80s fashion was ripe with Lady Diana–inspired shoulder pads, vivid colors, and lots of chunky costume jewelry to complete the look. Pushing accessories and special occasion dresses covered the extra money I needed to pay my rent. That night, as I exchanged pleasantries and sold boatloads of gold necklaces and silver earrings, I couldn't ignore the discomfort that pressed against my skin.

On Tuesday, I drove to the University District to explain my symptoms to a doctor. A nurse drew my blood and asked me to pee in a cup. Then I waited alone in an uncomfortable wooden chair propped against the wall and focused on the vinyl wallpaper and tiles—a study in beige on beige. The fluorescent fixtures hummed overhead, blanketing me in a harsh, artificial light. Windowless clinic rooms are never cheerful, but thankfully in my young life, I hadn't seen many. The doctor walked in and sat down at the little desk next to me.

He was tall and thin, with brown leather shoes that he undoubtedly chose for comfort over style. His face looked serious—no smile or friendly eye twinkle, and his white hair matched his white doctor's coat. He delivered his words softly, but they hit hard. "I'm sorry, young lady. The result indicates your kidneys are damaged."

I gave him a few seconds to tell me it was a joke, but he didn't seem like the jokester type, and come to think of it, how unfunny of a joke would *that* be? My mind raced with nonsensical thoughts. Yet this doctor was no-nonsense (his practical shoes . . . case in point), and this situation was the farthest thing possible from a joke.

I didn't realize at the time that these few moments with this unfamiliar man would forever link to the moment my life changed forever.

2.

Holes

HIS WORDS ECHOED IN MY MIND—*YOUR KIDNEYS ARE damaged, your kidneys are damaged*—as the walls seemed to fold in. *Is this room getting smaller?* "You will need to have a biopsy to determine the extent and cause of the damage," he explained. His eyes traversed from my newly created medical file to my stunned face.

"A biopsy?" *Isn't this a cancer word?* I fidgeted in my chair and stared at him like he was speaking a foreign language.

What happened to the standard doctor line? You have a simple case of (fill-in-the-blank) and I will prescribe (fill-in-the-blank) and voilà, better in three to four days. I'd take a cold, maybe the flu, a simple strep throat—one of those familiar ailments, please. But "biopsy" fell outside my medical comfort zone.

He said they'd found protein in my urine (officially known as proteinuria), which was causing the fluid retention. Protein has no place in urine. The tiny filters in healthy kidneys, the nephrons, do not allow protein to pass through, just as a coffee filter does not let coffee grounds pass into your coffee pot. My kidneys' nephrons were like a lousy coffee filter with holes. Microscopic holes. But still, I didn't yet realize the power of things I could not see.

"The biopsy will help us diagnose what's causing your kidneys to leak protein," he explained.

Right away, I called home. My mom booked the first flight from Minneapolis to Seattle. I learned later she'd experienced an immediate sinking feeling after my initial call three days earlier. She'd heard something in my voice, and ripples creased her tight-knit maternal fabric—she felt sure I was experiencing something far from the flu.

My parents urged me to have the biopsy in Minneapolis, my hometown, because my dad knew and trusted a nephrologist, Dr. David Brown. My dad built custom homes, and years earlier, he contracted a lovely place for Dr. Brown and his wife. But we'd never expected to seek Dr. Brown's expertise in kidney care.

Lisa sat by my side when I called Nick to tell him the news. He asked, "What are they looking for with a biopsy?" His voice shook.

"The cause of damage. I'm going to Minneapolis to find out what's going on, and then I'll be back for Sarah's party." Lisa stood to face me, cocked her sweatpants-clad hip, and widened her ice-blue eyes. (Sarah was another Seattle resident and college friend.)

"Jen," Lisa said, narrowing her gaze, "Sarah's party is not your top concern. It's in two weeks." Nick said the same thing, but two weeks seemed like a long time to me.

"Well, I better be on the mend by then," I suggested to Nick on the phone, to Lisa in the room, and to the Fix-It gods who may have been eavesdropping.

I had met Lisa in a freshman communications class. I sat directly behind her and focused on the back of her head. Her blond hair, the thickest golden mane I'd ever seen, became a visual distraction to the long lecture. She also picked her lower lip repeatedly, as if it helped her concentrate. We chatted after class and quickly became friends.

After college, Lisa and I lived for a short stint with our

friend Cindy in a duplex apartment in Seattle's Capitol Hill neighborhood. A cast of characters (hidden homeless men scared us silly when we'd hear, "Goodnight," as we walked past the nearby bushes) and a series of unfortunate events (a Peeping Tom and subsequent robbery) made us want to bolt out of there quickly. Cindy took a job with Pan Am to fly the friendly skies, and Lisa and I moved into the apartment close to the Space Needle on Queen Anne Hill.

Lisa's retail job suited her. She had a great sense of style (inherited from her mom, who sold clothing for couture designers) and preferred work she could leave behind at the end of the day. Hosiery wasn't her dream department, but she didn't miss the textbooks and tests of our college days. At night, after work, we donned sweatpants and ponytails, ate grocery store sushi, cracked open cans of Diet Orange Sunkist, and laughed out loud watching David Letterman.

The next day, I picked up my mom at the airport, and her Julie Andrews–esque auburn hair, fair complexion, and lovely countenance ushered in a familiar wave of safety. We stopped at the grocery store, picked up a few items, and headed home.

"Nice," Mom said when she took in our greige-stained wood floors and freshly painted walls. I showed off our new digs and set her suitcase in my room. After we unloaded the groceries into our spare cabinets and nearly empty refrigerator, she said, "You don't have any food. What do you girls usually eat?"

Lisa and I shared a glance. "Stuff that doesn't go in the oven," I replied, and we laughed. The three of us sat together at our little white hand-me-down card table (this was the first time we actually set the table too), and the Mom-made hot dinner nourished us.

"What do you think is going on?" Mom asked as she lowered a napkin to her lap.

"I don't know . . . it doesn't make sense. I eat healthy, I'm not into drugs—I even floss. Sometimes."

"Flossing is overrated," Lisa said. She smiled as she moved a chunk of her thick blond hair behind her ear. Mom laughed too, but when her smile faded, I saw a flash of concern flood her eyes. Later, she shared that when I greeted her at the airport, she knew her instincts were right. I was not well.

But for me, until this point, "not well" prompted Vitamin C or chicken soup for my soul. Quick fix. Move on. I thought that's how it always worked. I had a lot to learn. The next day, Mom and I flew to Minneapolis. It was late November 1987, and the chain of events had just begun.

3.

Punch

THE NEXT MORNING, I SPRAWLED FACEDOWN ON A STIFF, rolling bed in a sterile hospital room. While I waited for the procedure to begin, the thin blanket that covered me was no match for the cold circulating air. My muscles twitched.

While my parents sat together in the nearby waiting room, a nurse by my side shot a magic elixir into my IV, and within seconds the tense, frosty edges melted away.

Dr. Brown stood next to me. "How do you feel?" he asked.

"Floaty."

A squirt. Cold, slimy gel on my back. Dr. Brown explained he would place five tiny needles into one of my kidneys, guided by ultrasound. Afterward, we'd know more about why my kidneys leaked protein.

"You will feel pressure and hear a loud click from the needle punch," Dr. Brown said. His description was accurate. The pushing sensation was painless, but the sound startled me—as if a cap gun fired into my back.

"We've done one. Okay? Now we will do a couple more."

Push. Pressure. Punch. Click. Wince. Breathe.

Push. Pressure. Punch. Click. Wince. Breathe.

Push. Pressure. Punch. Click. Wince. Breathe.

Push. Pressure. Punch. Click. Wince. Breathe.

I could not believe this was happening. I was fine less than two weeks ago.

"We've got some good samples," Dr. Brown said. "Now we wait. I want you to stay on bed rest for twenty-four hours."

An attendant wheeled me from the procedure room, deep in the bowels of the hospital, up to my room on the fourth floor. A nurse placed sandbags on my back to prevent bleeding. As instructed, I lounged as still as possible, but my insides fluttered. *What the hell?*

Every story begins with a domino moment that starts a chain of events. My first domino had fallen.

I had common goals for my life at the time. As twentysomethings do. I planned to launch into a public relations career after my performance as a star intern. In my professional dealings along the way, or in my robust Pacific Northwest social circle, perhaps, I would meet a rom-com-worthy guy. A soulmate? Sure. He would be so rock-solid, so handsome, so irreverent—oh, the laughter and deep connections—that I would regularly think, *How can I be so lucky to have caught this guy?* (Though Nick and I had been dating for a few years, he wasn't the one I envisioned in this scenario.)

Mr. Perfect and I would live blissfully in a lovely and oh-so-happy home, where I'd whip together meals that would be today's version of Instagram food porn. And like a cherry on top, I'd pump out photogenic babies and display my perfect family on annual holiday cards. All the while, gracefully keeping it together as a how-does-she-do-it professional career woman. Nicely wrapped up and tied with a bow.

Well, maybe that is the amped-up and glossy version. But boiled to the essence, my peers and I expected to travel a path that led us into the epitome of adulthood—career, love, family. Up until this point, happy was my default setting; I'd never really considered an alternate state.

And now, plucked from the West Coast and Puget Sound, I

shivered in the frigid winter of Minnesota, in a hospital with Mom, Dad, Dr. Brown, and yet-to-be-understood kidney damage. The end of my twenty-second year spun off the path of grandiose expectations and careened right off a cliff.

4.

Limbo

MY PARENTS AND I HAD TO WAIT A WEEK FOR THE BIOPSY results. The window narrowed on Sarah's party, but I still entertained the idea. I returned to my parents' suburban home, where I had grown up with my older brother, Steve. My dad built this home for our family when I started kindergarten and Steve first grade. Like a two-story stationary time capsule made of gray wood siding, crisp white trim, and a gabled roof, it was chockfull of childhood memories.

I retreated into my childhood room, looked at my swollen ankles, and felt the pressure from the extra fluid invading my cells. *How sick am I?*

When my dad initially presented me with wallpaper options for this space, I chose pink and blue flowers, splattered delicately across a creamy white backdrop. I loved those flowers. A pink shag carpet (think Pepto-Bismol) added even more girly wow factor. An overflowing dollhouse and giant corkboard (pinned to the max with crayon pictures) completed my little heaven.

During my teenage years, primary colors replaced pastels. Bruce Springsteen concert stubs, images of Paris, and a magazine cover of Cindy Crawford (to inspire my perfect self) replaced elementary school art.

Pins pushed remnants of my teenage mindset into that cork because my mom wanted to keep the room inviting for holiday visits. It seemed both familiar and foreign, the younger, pre-adult version of me on that corkboard ready to say hi.

I called my Seattle friends and delivered the same update over and over: "Yes, I had the biopsy. No, I don't know anything. Waiting. Will let you know. How are you? Hoping to be back for Sarah's party. See you soon."

The following Monday, Mom, Dad, and I sat in the lobby of Dr. Brown's clinic. It appeared far more polished than the doctor's office in Seattle, and I stared trancelike at the bronze-toned wallpaper.

A nurse escorted us back to a clinic room. The hard edges of the plastic chair mirrored the discomfort of my mind and body. Dr. Brown sported a bow tie and tweed suit, greeted us curtly, and sat down. He adjusted round wire-rim glasses and ruffled through the pages in my chart.

My dad leaned forward on the edge of his chair like a take-charge CEO ready to tackle an issue. I saw a focused anticipation in his brown eyes. Coarse dark hair topped his round face, which made him look younger than his fifty-two years. My mom's eyes were deep wells of blue, reflecting worry. She rested her hand on mine. Dr. Brown set the papers on the desk and delivered six words: "You have a progressive kidney disease."

For a moment, I considered myself a character in a cheesy soap opera who gets bad news—the words reverberated inside my mind while my face registered a melodramatic pause. But I was not a character, and this was not a script.

Progressive disease.

Progressive disease.

Progressive disease.

What?

Dr. Brown explained a condition called nephrotic syndrome

was causing inflammation in the tiny filters of my kidneys. The three of us sat with dazed expressions as he continued to educate us about my problem. I was grateful to have my parents in the room because I had trouble focusing. As we sat together vested in my outcome, I felt like a middle school student receiving negative feedback at a teacher conference.

"The biopsy indicates focal segmental glomerulosclerosis."

"That's a mouthful," I said, stunned.

"Also known as focal sclerosis or FSGS," Dr. Brown explained.

"How does this happen?" Dad asked.

"Larry, I can't answer that. Jennifer has an autoimmune dysfunction, and we don't know the cause."

"Do you know the cure?" *An excellent question, Dad.* But the word itself seemed surreal. *Cure.* This was uncharted territory—sitting in a small clinic room conversing about a progressive disease that had afflicted me out of the blue.

"What we need to do now is monitor the kidneys and try to stop the damage with a medication called prednisone."

"Will prednisone fix it?" I asked. I wanted a simple answer and did not realize how complicated the question was.

Dr. Brown told us there is a child-onset nephrotic syndrome that responds well to treatment. "It's unclear, Jennifer, at twenty-two, if you are experiencing a late child-onset case, or if your case will be more advanced. I would like to consult with some colleagues and see you back here in a few days."

The child-onset route seemed the better of the two syndromes. So I pinned my hopes on having the kid version. That scenario could make this condition go poof and evaporate with prednisone. I planted this idea firmly in my mind.

Child onset. Please. Child onset.

I wasn't alone with this diagnosis, and my parents' concern somehow diluted my own. Deep in my inner-child self, I believed my parents could shield me from outside harm. Later, I'd learn the extensive truths and limits of that belief.

My childhood had been a regular one, filled with youthful things. I loved dolls, played T-ball (I was the pitcher—which is more like a pretend skill, you don't even have to pitch), ice-skated in the winter, made crafts with my Bluebird troop, made up elaborate stories, dashed around on my bike and skateboard, and sent Ping-Pong balls flying around the basement with my brother. There was a lot of normalness, and I desperately wanted to stay normal.

Steve and I grew up in a relatively drama-free household, but we had typical episodes of sibling rivalry. Being a fan of *The Brady Bunch*, I reacted to each big-brother injustice with Marcia-like theatrics. "It's not fair that I am penalized because I was born one year later!" I think I memorized this line from an episode and delivered it often with dramatic flair.

Drama seemed warranted a few times. Steve tossed my favorite doll, Peggy, overboard on a boating adventure. That was traumatic. He also flung the phone receiver at my head once. That was rude. The stuff of a big brother, but we were different kids for sure. Steve was rowdy, and I was obedient and approval seeking.

As youngsters, we had an occasional babysitter named Mrs. Sawyer. She was an older woman and pretty stern by my recollection. She teased her short gray hair (grandma style) and wore old-fashioned glasses with black topping the frame and gold around the rest. They weren't retro-cool frames on the austere Mrs. Sawyer, and I bet if she were a nun, she would have rapped knuckles with a ruler.

She branded me as the good girl, in contrast to Steve's rebellious ways. I sat quietly, coloring inside the lines with my box of sixty-four Crayola crayons, while Steve threw balls and Lincoln Logs all over the place. He didn't concern himself with obedience or approval, much to the chagrin of ole Battle-Ax Sawyer.

Her go-to discipline technique when things got out of hand involved the corner time-out. Steve was always the one forced to sit still in the designated chair. As he fumed, waiting for the release from his prison, Mrs. Sawyer would shake her head and proclaim, "I could take a thousand Jennifers, but only one Steve."

This might not seem to be a great babysitting technique, but the truth is, I liked that a lot. I always was a fan of pleasing people. And now, what I assumed would please everyone, more than anything, would be to relegate this disruptive illness to the corner and return to my trouble-free kid version of Jennifer.

The haziness of my initial diagnosis mirrored the confusing intersection of time and place in my life. I was not a child, nor was I perfectly positioned within adulthood—I hung in life-stage limbo—the space between reliance and independence. While forging my way into the post-college world, I hadn't yet put the last puzzle piece into place. Now the image of the puzzle had shifted into something else entirely.

Although I was far from my Seattle home, I had returned to a place where I knew I always fit. I was my parents' daughter. It became clear my mom and dad would swiftly join forces with me, like my private National Guard, to engage in disaster response.

I had trouble sleeping that evening, focusing on the goal of being an adult with a child's illness. I remembered when my mom used to tuck me in and wish me sweet dreams, way back when those wallpaper flowers surrounded me. With Steve one room away, our dog Gus asleep downstairs, and my parents nearby at the end of the hall, the world had seemed nothing but safe.

And now, unsettled, I tossed and turned and pulled up the window shade. Cold air wafted from the chilled panes of glass and hit my face. I looked at the November snow-covered landscape, a frozen version of Seattle rain, and hoped prednisone would bring me back to the place where I belonged.

I saw two outcomes to this situation. Heal or fail. I wanted to heal.

5.

Mortality?

AT MY FOLLOW-UP APPOINTMENT A FEW DAYS LATER, Dr. Brown said there was a consensus among his colleagues that prednisone should be the first course of treatment. Prednisone is an anti-inflammatory prescribed for a wide variety of ailments, from arthritis to asthma to poison ivy. It's a wonder drug, but a nasty beast in high doses. The list of side effects was bizarre and disturbing.

"You may feel extremely hungry, so be careful about gaining weight."

"Okay . . ."

"You can avoid weight gain if you are careful, but your cheeks will almost certainly puff into a moon face. Possibly your stomach too," he continued, like he had recited this script many times before. "Also, muscle wasting—skinny arms and skinny legs. Sticklike."

"Chipmunk cheeks and twiggy arms and legs?" I said in horror. "Sounds pretty bad."

Dr. Brown was not done. Weak bones. High blood pressure. High blood sugar. Cataracts. Insomnia. Rat-a-tat-tat. His delivery was flat and matter-of-fact. I was envisioning my upcoming disfigurement, my future as a strangely proportioned Fig Newton character, as he continued to tick off the side effects like a grocery list.

If this moment was superimposed on a modern-day pharmaceutical commercial, his warnings would be the voice-over while I walked jauntily on a sunshiny fairway, laughed over a missed putt, and enjoyed a most pleasant backdrop as the warning "Fat face, fat stomach, weak arms, weak legs, uncontrollable hunger, general onset of shitty life" narrated the picturesque scene.

"You're freaking me out," I said.

"I'd be remiss if I failed to mention the possibility of a personality change, Jennifer. You could become manic or anxious." He seemed committed to this thorough information delivery, like a lawyer covering all the liability bases.

"Is there another option?" I asked.

"No. This is our best option."

Oh, great. Sign me up, I thought with dismay.

There was no surefire treatment for FSGS, so I was confident this diagnosis fit into the dreaded and highly technical medical classification known as Big Bummer. Dr. Brown explained that a blood test would check my creatinine level, an important measure of kidney function. What glucose is for people with blood sugar issues, creatinine is for kidney patients. So he would continually monitor my creatinine and the amount of protein in my urine.

"How are you feeling?" he asked, scrutinizing my face like a museum painting.

"Swollen and tired. I don't have much energy, and I don't pee much."

He nodded. "I'm not surprised. The protein leak is why you are retaining fluid. Let's start on the prednisone and see how you do." Dismal side effects aside, I was motivated to take anything to rid my body of the proteinuria and kidney damage.

Bring it on, prednisone. I started taking it every morning. With each round white pill I swallowed, I set my intention upon closing that protein leak and returning to my apartment in Seattle with Lisa. Sarah's party, however, had come and gone.

Now I hunkered down in Golden Valley, Minnesota, with two jobs: 1) take prednisone as prescribed and 2) wait until I got better. I had notified Stacy that I wouldn't be back to complete my internship, and the lost opportunity felt like a robbery.

The first thing I noticed from the pill popping was the insane energy level—imagine the Energizer Bunny fueled with a quadruple espresso. There was no closet I didn't attempt to clean or shelf of books I didn't want to alphabetize.

"Mom, I think this prednisone will do it," I said one morning as I sat down at the kitchen table with a mug of tea. I had about seven days of prednisone coursing through my system, and although I feared the medication might not work, I refused to say it out loud as if airing the thought could jinx my healing.

"Me too," she said, and sat down by my side with her cup of coffee in hand. As we gripped our hot beverages, I looked beyond the French doors to a vacant bird feeder that hung from a leafless tree branch. The birds had flown south for the winter. Lucky birds. It was cold, and I felt tethered to Minnesota; I envied their freedom.

"I want to learn more," I said. If there was anything besides prednisone that would help, I wanted to jump on it.

"Should we do research?" Mom asked. "We could go to the biomedical library." (This was pre-Internet. Now it's hard to imagine that libraries used to be the go-to source for information.)

My mom had raised me before various labels categorized parenting (helicopter, free-range, tiger); she just lovingly dove into the nooks and crannies of my every day with enthusiasm. I'd looked forward to the fourth-grade Fridays when she volunteered at my school and puffed with pride when other kids said, "Your mom is so nice."

When a frustrated boy threw a phonics book at her and the kids in the class were all abuzz, she skillfully diffused the moment by distracting us and keeping the room calm. She had been an elementary school teacher before Steve and I were born, and she knew how to practice patience amid chaos.

She learned to play the piano along with Steve and me (we took lessons) and became my duet partner during the recital at our teacher's house. Together, we tinkered it out, a plucky version of "Come Saturday Morning."

Everything was better with her hand—homework, holidays, and hamburgers. Books and library visits were right up her alley too, so our medical library adventure would seem reminiscent of what we'd done when I was a kid.

Later that day, Mom and I made our way east on I-94 to the vast University of Minnesota campus, parked in the closest lot, and hustled down Delaware Street. Bundled up in down jackets, we scurried against the wind and entered the Phillips-Wangensteen Building, the home of the biomedical research library. With tote bags filled with notebooks, pens, and pencils, we were researchers on a mission.

The librarian led us to stacks of medical publications with FSGS research—*Kidney International, The American Journal of Kidney Diseases,* and *The New England Journal of Medicine.*

"We scored," I said to my mom as we plopped many publications on a long wooden table. We didn't understand what we were looking for, but a surplus of helpful information was indexed and ours for the reading.

"Let's dive in," Mom said in a quiet library voice, and buried her nose in a technical article. We became fellow researchers on a quest to unlock the mystery of my sudden diagnosis. But as we tried to decipher complicated kidney research, we quickly realized we had inadequate backgrounds to comprehend the information.

Technical, written in nephrology code, most of it went right over our heads.

"Do you understand what you're reading?" Mom asked.

"A little between the lines." Statistical references and timelines for morbidity and mortality wove throughout the difficult text. "Must say I'm not loving the stuff about FSGS mortality rates." These words pinched me, so I skipped over them and didn't look at the numbers.

Much later, I searched the Internet for this information again and read a 1978 abstract from *Clinical Nephrology* that studied the long-term prognosis of forty FSGS patients between the span of six to sixteen years. A decade after this study began, eleven patients had normal kidney function, eight patients had compromised kidney function, and the remaining twenty-one patients were deceased, on dialysis, or transplanted. I didn't want to pollute my thoughts with statistics on the front end of my diagnosis, however; I was too young and invincible to consider my mortality. So I didn't.

I developed a Teflon coating for my mind. Words like *morbidity* slid away. I didn't deny I had a health problem; obviously, that's why we were there. I just refused to fold frightening statistics into my brain; I knew nothing about the conditions of the people who comprised those numbers, except that they were not me.

"Maybe this is too much," my mom said. Her face drained of color in the dim overhead lighting.

"No, it's okay. There's some good stuff here," I said. Sure, I understood little of what I read. But this library excursion was more of an empowerment event—reading complicated medical journals felt like taking a stand against our invader. And I say *our* invader because that's how my mom made me feel. Like this was ours to battle together.

I left the library with a sense of having accomplished something. That's the thing about using hope to fuel action—no matter how small, it still feels like action. I set out to do whatever it took. I wanted to live.

6.

Manifest

LISA AND THE OTHER THREE IN OUR POSSE, CINDY, SUSAN, and Gillian, kept me up-to-date on all the Seattle parties I missed, the new jobs people landed, and the new boyfriends snagged. I was grateful for the updates, but I couldn't help feeling envious each time our conversations ended. Their lives advanced while mine stalled.

Nick had moved to London to complete his final credits in a study abroad program, and although we wrote letters, we'd decided to take a break while he was gone.

I'd always liked the way Nick made me feel—my jokes made him laugh, and he doted on me. We told each other everything about everything. Like best friends, we laughed a huge percentage of the time, danced freely at parties, and wore our relationship like a favorite pair of jeans. Go-to. Good fit. Comfy. Still, I didn't know if we had a forever thing going, so our break became a welcome test.

Boy was I lonely, though. I felt utterly isolated being back in Minneapolis. It didn't help that my high school friends had scattered throughout the country after graduation. But I knew I had some healing to attend to, and even if my friends were home, I wouldn't be up for going out with gusto.

After several weeks of ingesting loads of prednisone, my face plumped up like an overfilled balloon. The dreaded moon-face effect was underway. I stared at myself in the mirror in disbelief.

One evening, I curled up on the couch with a throw blanket

to ease my constant chilliness (another side effect of compromised kidneys) as my dad arrived home from work.

"I got you something," he said, tossing me a bag. I pulled out a hardcover book, *Love, Medicine, and Miracles.*

"Thanks, Dad," I said as I studied the back cover. The author, Dr. Bernie S. Siegel, a surgeon, recounted his personal experiences with ill patients. He found that stress reduction, attitude shifts, and "taking control" of illness positively impact the outcome.

Not long before, this book wouldn't have stood out to my dad in the bookstore. But now his daughter was a sick girl in search of love, medicine, and miracles. How quickly our entire world had changed. But I felt determined to beat this.

I smiled. "This might do the trick, Dad."

I devoured the book. Published in 1986, the many patient recovery stories inspired my mental mission to take control and heal. Success or failure was in my court, and I wanted to ace the healing curriculum like a stellar student. It was attainable. Dr. Bernie Siegel said so. He had seen cases of self-healing from "exceptional patients."

Apparently, the answer to healing hinged upon my ability to be an "exceptional patient." No pressure.

Dad cheered me on, and it was a job that suited him well. His eager, wide-eyed look complimented his persona as a positive-thinking advocate; his expression invited action. For years Dad would quote Dale Carnegie, author of *How to Win Friends and Influence People*, at the dinner table for Steve and me, while my mom rolled her eyes. It was my dad's version of the family Bible. WWDD: What would Dale do?

His favorite Carnegie book, *How to Stop Worrying and Start Living*, espoused the basic stop-worry concept Dad promoted. "Think of the worst thing that could happen to you with any situation, and accept it," Dad had explained.

He mentioned this concept to me again as we waited to see if the prednisone was working. Sitting at the kitchen table, I said, "That sounds too simple, plus I can think of some pretty bad things, Dad."

"Dale (note the first-name basis) says if you can *prepare* yourself to accept the worst, and then actually improve upon this scenario, the hard part is done. Then worry can't overtake you." Dad motioned with his arms as he preached his philosophy, a sure sign he believed it was important. This worry-reduction technique was effective for him as a builder because he had to withstand many economic ups and downs in the volatile construction industry. His strategy was to accept the possibility of failure to clear the way for success.

"Yeah, but then I'd have to think about the prednisone not working, and I can't bring myself to think about that," I said. I looked down and traced the edges of my place mat.

"I don't blame you, Jenny," he replied. His face softened. I think my words reminded him we weren't talking about the success or failure of a business. "Let's focus on everything being okay."

"That I can do." I half smiled, relieved to be off the hook of going down the accept-the-worst path just yet. *Everything will be okay. Everything will be okay.*

Dad had developed tools to navigate life. Before this, I hadn't faced momentous struggles that required life tools. Dad's ideas led me through the back door of positive thinking and taught me to believe I could set my course through thoughts and action. Dr. Siegel's book reinforced this idea as well.

Dad had taught Steve and me to be tough against mild ailments. If we asked to stay home from school because of something minor, he challenged the idea with unusual stories of perseverance. One of our favorites (and God only knows where he got this one) was about a guy that "played baseball with a hole in his arm." So apparently, even if we woke up with a hole in our arm, Dad would encourage us to be brave and learn about algebra anyway. How does one get a hole in the arm? This remains a mystery, but the point was taken.

Dad's perseverance pep talks did not alter Steve's accident-prone nature, mixed with some early health scares. There was the time my brother split his lip from a poorly thrown Magic 8 Ball (not a great throwing toy). There was the broken-bone Ping-Pong injury when his friend Freddy tossed the paddle at Steve's hand. And during elementary school, Steve suffered from severe headaches. They prompted neurological tests, a series of hospitalizations, and a middle-of-the-night rush to the operating room. An appendectomy followed. In contrast, I sailed through my youth without a stitch, a broken bone, or a hospital stay.

After Steve graduated from college in upstate New York, he moved to Philadelphia. My college years in Washington State situated me on the other side of the country. Now he was twenty-three to my twenty-two and had snagged a job and an apartment on the East Coast. I had not seen him for several months, but we chatted on the phone.

Dad never brought up that crazy hole-in-the-arm story in the face of migraines, a ready-to-burst appendix, and sudden autoimmunity. But years later, I would realize his underlying message was a helpful guide—no matter what, keep going.

Meanwhile, Mom and I continued to seek ammunition for my healing arsenal, so we went to a New Age bookstore in Minneapolis. As we pushed past split-beaded entry curtains, the musky aroma of burning incense struck us. It couldn't have been more different from the biomedical library. Underfoot was a faded, well-worn Persian rug, and many shelves offered a treasure trove of books. Perhaps these pages contained the secret to crack the healing code?

We smelled varieties of incense, tasted samples of herbal teas, and homed in on authors who illuminated visualization techniques. Again, hope-fueled action took place in a space filled with books. We left with a paperback, *Creative Visualization*, by Shakti Gawain. The pages promised affirmations to guide me toward what I wanted in my life.

I could not put this book down. Each page pulled me into the laws of attraction, a concept I had felt intuitively, perhaps, but never with such clarity and magnetic appeal. *Love, Medicine, and Miracles* drew the lines, and *Creative Visualization* filled them in. These books were a timely pair to inspire the idea that my mind could attract what I wanted. Several times a day, and before I went to sleep at night, I envisioned my triumphant return to Seattle with restored health.

I didn't realize then that mind-body imagery and positive affirmations would provide lifelong tools for me, as Dale Carnegie did for Dad. I would continue to use these resources in the upcoming decades to direct my thoughts, help me let go, and learn to live.

My mom's dedication to join my pursuit of healing and my dad's positivity (and books to back it up) compounded into a potent medicine. I knew if their big dose of love could have eradicated my ailment, it would have. But I'd started to learn about the stronger forces beyond the reach of powerful parental love.

7.

Hide

WHEN I SWALLOWED MY DAILY PILLS, I IMAGINED prednisone dissolving into my bloodstream like a pharmaceutical superhero hell-bent on destroying my inflammation. Dr. Brown had mentioned that sometimes nephrotic syndrome resolves from spontaneous remission. That sounded good to me. And so I focused on manifesting it day and night. *Spontaneous remission. Spontaneous remission. Spontaneous remission. Please? Pretty please?* I recited this intention and imagined a healing golden light encircling my pink kidneys.

Toward the end of December, Steve came home for Christmas. We reminisced about when we used to bound downstairs at the crack of dawn to unwrap the bounty that Santa had squeezed down the chimney. That was when we'd believed in the miracle of a red-suited, white-bearded man with magical gift-delivery skills.

Our family of four attended Christmas Mass together. This service was an obligatory family outing, but I was content to fold into the collection of voices singing familiar songs. Growing up, we attended a progressive Catholic church that welcomed people of all faiths. We sat in folding chairs in a school gymnasium, a very un-churchy setting, and listened to thought-provoking speakers. It felt more like a humanistic PBS hour than it did a devout religious experience, and I liked the engaging speakers and music.

As Steve and I became teenagers, our church attendance dwindled down to holidays, and I didn't seek any religious experiences during college. The contemplation of higher powers hadn't made it to the top of my list yet. My spiritual awareness lay dormant.

When my extended family gathered at my parents' home for the Christmas meal this year, I avoided eye contact with my aunts, uncles, and cousins. The swelling in my face inflated my self-consciousness, and I felt their curious gazes bore into me. I had yet to learn that what felt like pity was concern and kindness.

Dr. Brown explained prednisone causes chipmunk cheeks because it rearranges the fat in your body. I felt like this medication altered every ounce of me. He also prescribed diuretics to help eliminate the fluid retention. My fluid-obscured, young-person-old-lady ankles hurt, and my eyes still burrowed into marshmallow-like eye sockets. My face tingled; I swear I could feel the prednisone shuffling fat to my cheeks.

I became convinced the big-cheek side effect would stop if I cut out all fat from my diet. I wanted to beat the system and gain some sense of control. Besides low-fat foods, Dr. Brown prescribed a low-protein diet to reduce the stress on my kidneys.

My daily routine consisted of black tea with low-protein toast and jam for breakfast, low-sodium vegetable soup and low-protein crackers for lunch, and a half of a baked potato with vegetables for dinner. I monitored my food intake obsessively, as if my life depended on it—well, in my defense, it did.

I went upstairs and stared at myself in the bathroom mirror. My eyes pulled wide-open and my cheeks sucked in, I tried to see a resemblance to my old self. *Maybe it's not that bad?* While brushing my hair, the bristles clogged with long, loose strands. *My hair can't be falling out.* I kept brushing. The loose hair kept coming. I continued brushing and brushing, thinking I could get rid of the loose hair and that would be the end of it. But there was no end.

Oh no. I am losing everything. It felt like a slow-motion fall into a chasm. I wanted to hide in a hole until I could crawl out as the old me. It didn't occur to me I might never return to that version of myself.

8

Crystal

THOUGHTFUL CARDS FLOODED THE MAILBOX. GILLIAN, A college friend who worked as a Seattle elementary school teacher, asked her class to draw pictures to cheer up her sick friend. She sent me a packet filled with crayon artwork. My favorite was a stick figure in a bed, a square box for the mouth, and red crayon hair that stood straight up. Above the electrocuted-looking figure was a scribbled caption, "Yur Pretty."

Mom's friends dropped off baskets with bath salts and lotions. More books. And novelty tokens of warm wishes, such as an envelope labeled "Fairy Dust" with a drawing of an angel. I put that envelope by my bed and referred to it as my angel dust.

Kindness bowled me over, but I didn't yet know these gestures only skimmed the surface. Later, I learned the depth to which people's big-heartedness would extend.

"Jenny?" I heard my mom calling me from downstairs. "Rachael's on the phone." Rachael and I grew up together, fully intertwined throughout middle and high school. I picked up the line.

"How are you doing?" Rachael asked in her endearing, nasal-toned voice, which ignited my intense longing for better times. Just as Christmas with Steve rekindled memories of youthful innocence, Rachael's voice reminded me of silly conversations about boy crushes, makeup lessons, and passing notes in class. I felt homesick for unencumbered, health-free thoughts. "I'm in town, hon, and I want to see you."

"Well . . . I don't look good, so it's not a great time," I said, glancing down at my sausage-like fingers. I grimaced as the fluid pressure stretched the skin on my shins and feet. "The medication is playing some nasty tricks on me. Let's wait until some side effects go away."

"That's ridiculous!" she declared. "I don't give a shit how you look. I want to see *you*."

I was lonely and missed Rachael in a huge way, but I wasn't *me*. Rachael wouldn't accept no, thank goodness, and visited the next day. Mom greeted her warmly at the door, but I approached sheepishly.

"Hi, honey, you look good," she said, giving me a big bear hug. Even if she didn't mean it, her sweetness relaxed me, and we sat down together in the family room. "I've got something for you," she said, and presented a clear, cylinder-shaped crystal.

"Ah, Rae, it's so pretty." I held the crystal up to the light.

"It allows positive energy to flow in and negative energy to flow out. It's healing," she explained.

"Love it! Let the healing begin!" I held it in my left hand and ran my right index finger along the side to absorb the positivity. I pulled away quickly. "Oh, it's a little sharp." I lifted my hand to see blood dripping from my finger.

"Oh Gawd," she said, her eyes expanding. But when she saw it was just a slight cut, she giggled. "Maybe we should set that down and try something else." Her little giggle took on steam and exploded into her characteristic, infectious, full-blown cackle.

Rachael's laugh is one of my favorite things in this world. It's a peal of laughter that spreads like wildfire. This was no exception, her laugh combining with the irony of the healing gift that drew blood, became hoots and howls that doubled us over.

When I could speak again, I asked, "You bring any other gifts?" Residual laughter upturned the corners of my lips, and I said, "How about a healing machete?"

Rae's cackle exploded again, and we laughed another round. Amid unexpected circumstances and sharp edges, laughter was the great normalizer. And I realized that despite my altered appearance, I was still me (sort of), and Rae was my friend. Avoiding love and support from loved ones was counterproductive, and I'd learn this repeatedly in the months and years to come.

9.

Perfection

DESPITE MY ATTEMPTS AT STAYING POSITIVE, LOSING MY
hair left me despondent and challenged the perfectionist in me.
The microscopic autoimmune factor in my blood remained invisible, and even the swelling in my face and ankles could go un-
noticed by people who didn't know me. But hair loss was entirely
different, the undeniable, final knockout. My takedown would
be apparent to everyone outside the ring, and the announcer
could call the fight. Sick girl, down.

I called Lisa to unload about my latest side effect. What was
she to say? So we did a conversational dance around it. Maybe it
will stop falling out. If not, go for a Sinead O'Connor look—we
bantered to buffer the situation. Thinking back, I know we both
resorted to lightness because the load became heavy. We were so
young to transition from watching *Cheers*, finding our first
apartments, and dealing with department store bosses to the
abrupt onset of life-changing illness.

While hair loss was an outward sign of my compromised
health, it also stoked old insecurities about where I fell on the
prettiness scale. I think my youthful adoration for *Charlie's Angels*
booted up this folly back in seventh grade. Two friends and I
would run around the neighborhood, hide behind trees, and pop
out with extended fake-gun arms and shout, "Freeze!" We gave
each other character assignments. I was Jaclyn Smith's Kelly. But
I really wanted to be Farrah. That hair!

As a brown-haired, freckle-faced, fourteen-year-old kid on course to top out at five feet, four inches (well, five feet, four and a half inches if I've done Pilates), I was so far from Farrah. But could I be better? Babysitting money in pocket, I rode my bike to the nearby corner drugstore to buy QT, the spray-tan equivalent of the day. I wanted to remedy my fair skin with a desirable bronze glow. The result?

Bronze? No.

Orange? Yes.

I also bought Sun-In, the spray-on hair product to provide a sun-kissed, California vibe while I hunkered down in snowy Minnesota. The result on brunette locks? Again, orange. *Very* orange.

I was figuring out how to fit into the world. Being pretty and pleasing seemed a worthy goal. From the youngest age, we slather praise on girls in the currency of "pretty"—*what a pretty dress, what pretty eyes, what pretty hair*. The "pretty" seeds planted in the fertile soil of my young mind sprouted perfectionism.

To be clear, let me define what I mean by perfectionism. I don't mean it in the clever job-interview-response way, as in: "What is your biggest weakness?" "My perfectionism!" It has nothing to do with the belief that everything I do is perfect, but the reverse. Everything I do is not even close.

In fact, I cringe to even use the p-word, fearing it will elicit criticism for how far I depart from perfect. But that's the problem. It's like having an impossible-to-please boss living inside your head who sets unattainable standards or goals, berates you for not measuring up, discourages you from taking risks, and chips away at your confidence.

So my preteen focus on angel-like looks layered a beauty-ideal over an established foundation of agreeability. And Mrs. Sawyer wasn't the only one who focused on my "goodness." My first-grade teacher, Mrs. McCarthy, who taught Steve the year before, told me I was a much easier student than my brother. Her comment took root.

"Easier."

Mrs. McCarthy and the angelic private detective show merged—sit quietly, don't ruffle feathers, and be a pretty little thing. I was a perceptive student of the messages that surrounded me. Today we are more mindful of the prevalent, limiting praise that encourages girls to speak at lower volumes, and encourage young girls, young women, and all women to speak up and be heard.

That seventh-grade, glamorous, finger-gun-toting (seems so inappropriate today) "angel" fantasy was behind me. Yet my per-sonality set like gelatin into the form of fitting in and pleasing people. This played into my attraction to Nick.

College was more difficult for him, so I helped him complete assignments. He elevated me to savior status when I spit out papers he'd struggled to write. I also listened with a sympathetic ear to stories of his complicated relationship with his father. He relied on me to help him gain perspective when he became overwhelmed. So I frequently shared my twentysomething life philosophy: Everything always works out in the end. I had every reason to put my full faith in that breezy belief. Nothing terrible had happened yet.

Nick was chatty. Fun. Entertaining. He thought I was smart. With strong legs, an athletic build, and honey-colored hair, he stopped me in my tracks with his blue-eyed gaze. Plus, he professed I was the only one who understood him. When he hoisted me onto a pedestal, I liked the view from up there.

Besides all that, he liked my hair. And now it was clogging my hairbrush in a mass exodus.

I still held on to the idea things would work out in the end.

But I welcomed the distance between Nick and me. Because seeing him would remind me of how far I'd traveled from my position on a pedestal. From my perfectionistic ideal. From my college days. From my healthy, wholesome, happy self.

10.

Riot

LISA AND I CONTINUED TO TALK ON THE PHONE, AND IN February, she rightfully and gingerly asked, "Are you coming back?" She had been living alone since November.

With conviction, I said, "Yes. I am. I just need a little more time, but I'll keep sending my share of the rent." My parents provided this share; I didn't have a job anymore, so they bridged these payments. They were eager to help, but even so, I felt enormous guilt.

I withstood a mounting load of indebtedness for everything they offered me, financially, emotionally, logistically, and wholeheartedly. Without the backup of my parents, my situation would have been significantly more unmanageable. I juggled guilt with immense gratitude as I appreciated my family.

"Get better, Jen," Lisa said with equal parts hope and heaviness. I felt determined that I would. Yet by spring, when tulips popped their cheerful reentry into the world, more fluid weighed my legs down. To walk, I had to drag them along with me.

I never appreciated my kidneys until they failed me. All the pints and gallons of blood they filtered, all the diet pops and coffee and iced tea they converted into urine. All the cheap Gallo Rhine wine they encountered when Lisa and I "pre-functioned" before fraternity parties. All the water they flushed through my system, all the potassium they cleared from vegetables, fruits, yogurt, and potatoes—all in the course of an ordinary twenty-four hours. My healthy pink kidneys did so much, continuously. I had never focused on their value.

But now I did.

I was due for a follow-up visit with Dr. Brown. Mom geared up for every appointment as a desirable social invitation and cheerfully referred to each one as a "riot." So when I asked if she wanted to come along, she said, "Love to! What a riot!"

"Checking in." I approached Teresa at the reception desk. Like always, she smiled and offered a warm welcome. Behind her were reams of color-coded files. File after file represented compromised kidney after compromised kidney. And they looked so neat. But I knew the files were tidy representations of untidy lives. Winners of the kidney lottery like me occupied a position in that file cabinet.

I took a seat next to my mom and grabbed a *People* magazine. Who among us doesn't appreciate flipping through *People* in a doctor's waiting room? Celebrity distraction pulled me back up to the surface from the bummer of those files. My mom read a book. I interrupted her reading with famous-people tidbits with no relevance to our lives. She feigned mock interest.

"Hey, Jennifer, come on back," Carol, my favorite nurse, said as she popped out to get me. With eager eyes and a toothy smile, she beamed like a friendly hostess welcoming me to her party. I liked her sparkle. Who says you can't have fun at a doctor's appointment? Misery doesn't need to drench every second, says I.

"How are you?" she asked after she recorded my weight and directed me to a side room. As the blood pressure cuff squeezed my arm, I answered, "I'm squishy." It seemed the best description because a push from my finger left a dent in my lower leg. My cheeks had ballooned from the prednisone.

"Squishy, I'll put that in your chart," she teased. "Hmm . . .

your weight's up. Your blood pressure's up. Have you been peeing?"

"Not much," I told her. I knew it wasn't normal, but I didn't know if it was an expected effect from my medication.

"Well, let's see what Dr. Brown says. He'll be in shortly."

Dr. Brown came in and shook my hand. I found his fussy formality endearing. He sat at the desk with his professorial manner, adjusted his glasses, and studied my chart. I saw him as a unique melding of Paul Simon, the singer, with Sherlock Holmes, the sleuth. In a good way. He oversaw my life, and there was no one else I wanted to be on my case. "How do you feel?" he asked as he rolled his chair toward me.

"I'm really puffy. Is this normal?" I said, extending my leg in the air to reveal my nonexistent anklebone.

He pressed down on my lower calf with his thumb, crumpled his brow, and crinkled his nose as if he smelled a skunk. "It could be from prednisone or disease progression. Tomorrow morning, I'd like you to start a twenty-four-hour urine collection, and we'll measure the spilled protein. After we compare it to your previous results, we'll know if the prednisone is helping."

"What's next?" my mom asked as we descended the elevator to the parking garage.

"Tomorrow I will be beholden to this." I held up a big brown jug and gave it a flick.

"Not fair, you get all the good stuff," my mom joked.

"Jenny and her jug. It's a great story."

Although we chuckled, we knew the results would be significant. Was I getting any better?

11.

Tangled

"JENNIFER, DR. BROWN HERE. THE RESULTS ARE BACK."
Gripping the phone, I squeezed my eyes shut, bracing for the
news. "I'm afraid the prednisone dose is not working. You are
spilling a larger quantity of protein."

"A lot more?" I asked. Every muscle in my body stiffened.

"Yes. A lot more. Massive proteinuria. I think we need to go
for broke," he said.

"What does that mean?"

"It's worth increasing the prednisone to four times a day.
That's a heavy dose, but we need to see if this will reduce the inflammation in your kidneys. We won't know unless we try," he
said softly.

I never questioned Dr. Brown's care. My parents and I put all
our faith in him. And the times were so different back then. I
couldn't consult Dr. Google and go down the rabbit hole of
searches to uncover FSGS treatments. I had a doctor, and he
knew best.

A heavy metal plate fell from my throat to my toes. I looked
up at the ceiling and took an audible breath. My mom came into
the kitchen and sat down on the edge of the chair next to me.
Still holding the phone, I looked at her and shook my head to
signal bad news. "Will the side effects get even worse?" I asked
Dr. Brown. My voice broke.

"Yes," he said. Of course they would. I don't even know why

I asked. "Remember," he continued, "the side effects are temporary. We are trying to save your kidneys here. That's most important."

Yes, yes, yes. I knew that. His words overwhelmed me. It was easier to focus on the physical changes to my appearance than on the underlying problem, the hidden inflammatory factor that circulated in my blood and damaged the tiny filters of my kidneys. A healthy kidney has about one million of these filters, and my rare disease was hell-bent on scarring segments of mine.

"Dr. Brown, how long will I be on this dose?" I asked. My shaky voice came out high and tight.

"As long as you can tolerate it."

"And what if it doesn't work?" I asked, trembling.

"Your kidneys may stop working, and if that happens, we'll have to consider dialysis and a kidney transplant." Dr. Brown was the expert, but I knew nothing about dialysis. So, dear reader, if you're unfamiliar, a dialysis machine is used to filter a patient's blood after their kidneys fail. Dialysis patients typically receive treatments at an outpatient clinic (or at home) between three to five times a week, for approximately three to four hours each time.

But healthy kidneys remove toxins twenty-four hours a day, seven days a week. When they fall down on the job, a dialysis machine is a part-time replacement for a full-time position.

I knew nothing about kidney transplants either. And my only experience with surgery was getting my wisdom teeth yanked out when I was sixteen. It wasn't pleasant because after returning home with Mom and Aunt Lucy, a thunderstorm knocked out the electricity. My plan to lounge on floor pillows, watch television, and eat ice cream was shot. But unnecessary teeth and vital organs were two very different things.

In my youthful view, a transplant seemed like a dramatic

movie-of-the-week topic, not something that would ever have to do with me. It seemed far-fetched and freaky. I didn't know that doctors had performed the first successful kidney transplant only thirty-five years earlier, in 1954. I didn't know that the field of transplantation had to reckon with the body's natural rejection response. I didn't know that only four years earlier, in 1983, the introduction of an immunosuppressant medication, cyclosporine, would inhibit the rejection response. And why would I?

It all seemed like so much to think about, so I clung to the idea that prednisone would work. "Okay, Dr. Brown, I'll pick up the new prescription today."

Before we finished the call, Dr. Brown said he wanted to see me in his clinic in two weeks. Mom sat eagerly by my side and waited for me to fill her in. "He's going to hammer me with more prednisone," I said.

"He is?" she said, in that oh-no kind of way. Her body collapsed a little, making her look smaller.

"I'm not sure how much my body can take." I wrung my hands, looked down, and fought back tears. "He mentioned dialysis and a transplant if it doesn't work."

Mom's face drained of color. I wished my body wasn't doing this to us. She didn't deserve to be a mom with a kidney-compromised kid. Steve called, and Mom told him the news. When she handed me the phone, Steve said, "Maybe it will work, Jenny."

"Maybe." All I could think about was the clobbering dose of the nasty drug.

"Don't worry, bodies can take a lot," Steve encouraged. "Take Eric Clapton, for example. He abused heavy drugs for years—major heroin addict. Look at him now. He looks great."

"Good point. I'm going to get pounded by prescription drugs, and rock on." And yet, I wondered, would I ever look "great" again? How well would my body withstand this?

And so it began, the big affair with prednisone. Four times a day. Swallowing the pills. Feeling holes rip through my stomach. Swigging Maalox to reduce the raging fire inside my gut to a constant burn.

Although extreme hunger is a common prednisone side effect, the reverse held true for me. My appetite vanished, but I had to eat something every time I swallowed one of those motherf**kers.

No.

No.

No.

Please, let this work. I had to heal. My visualizations continued. Several times each day and night, I conjured emerald lights dancing around my kidneys, a golden sun warming me and lifting me into a restored place of health and normalcy, and a smooth forward flow into my life ahead.

Within weeks after the increased dose, my hair became straggling wisps, like a young woman's version of Ebenezer Scrooge. It looked absurd, so I covered it with a scarf. My arms atrophied to skin and bone. My legs swelled so I could hardly walk. I couldn't wear any of my shoes. My cheeks pumped up like Gary Coleman's "Wha'choo you talkin' bout Willis?" (Mr. Coleman had kidney disease, and his signature chipmunk cheeks resulted from prednisone.)

Dr. Brown kept a close eye on my situation. My creatinine and proteinuria were both going in the wrong direction. Up. "I'm still worried about my legs," I told him at my two-week follow-up appointment, and showed him my no-ankle-bone ankle. Again, he extended my leg and pressed in with his thumb. The impression was so deep you could jam a few marbles in there.

I had complained to him about the fluid for a while, and

previously he wasn't that concerned. He expected fluid retention. But on this day, he said enough was enough.

"This is extreme. You don't have to walk around with this much fluid, Jennifer. I'd like to admit you for albumin transfusions and IV Lasix." The albumin would draw the extra fluid from my cells, and the high dose of the diuretic, Lasix, would help my struggling kidneys pee it away.

This plan excited me. Maybe I'd feel my legs again. Maybe I'd return to normal again. Maybe I'd look like me again. I went home, packed a bag with basics, and we headed to Abbott Northwestern Hospital with my mom.

My nurse, Katie, greeted me like an old friend. "Sorry to see you back here." I remembered her from my biopsy visit. "Here's a gown, robe, and socks. I'll leave them on the bed for you," she said.

"Katie, this isn't a great look for me. Do you have anything more tailored in a violet or rose shade?" I teased.

"Sure. I'll get our gown designer on it. But until then, this will have to do." She laughed. I begrudgingly tied on the dignity-stripping hospital gown, covered up with the robe, and plopped over the plastic side rails into the bed. The attire may have been lackluster, but the bed? Fabulous. The adjustability! Prop the head, elevate the feet, and the perfect television-watching position is a few up and down buttons away.

I had the power of a queen in this bed, a self-contained haven where my fingertips controlled all my whims and needs. The built-in television remote complete with lighting controls proved convenient. And with another button, I could buzz a request. A cold beverage, perhaps? More pillows? If it weren't for the needle sticks and continuous infusion of orange albumin, this could masquerade as something delightful!

Or so I tried to convince myself. So I chatted with my nurse and buoyed myself despite the hospitalization. I set out to be a cheerful brand ambassador for my case. *This isn't so bad.* Later, I realized how hard I tried to shine brightly in dim places.

After I settled in, a nurse placed an IV in my lower right arm. My mom claimed the chair in the corner and alternated between reading her book and cracking me up. Keeping things light was her specialty too, and I appreciated it. She also kept everything tidy, as though the order in this small space would expedite my hoping-to-heal body.

"Can I get you anything?" Mom asked as she walked over to the side of my bed and smoothed out the rumpled blankets. She became a human version of an accessible call button.

"No, thanks. I'm good," I said, turning my head toward her and readjusting the pillow. The albumin hung from an adjustable steel pole near the head of the bed, and a saline bag hung alongside it.

Mom wheeled the unwieldy, rolling pole and stepped closer to rearrange items on the table that overhung my bed. She moved the pole and turned to toss trash. She straightened the food tray, moved the pole again, and twisted to throw away another empty container. Somehow, she became tangled in the complex intersection of plastic tubes.

"Minor problem here," she said as she wrestled her way free (ever so gently) from the maze of tubing. She resembled Lucille Ball trying to keep up with the conveyor belt, wide-eyed, zany, determined. And adorable. It amused me as she navigated her way out of this comic mishap, trying to avoid tugging a line. We were living out our own medical sitcom, another fine mess, as we laughed through the tangled lines in my tangled life.

That evening, alone in my room, my cheerfulness lacked an audience, and my thoughts ran rampant in the dark. A frozen grip tightened my entire body. *What if this water weight is permanent? What if my kidneys are beyond repair?* I heard a commotion outside the room, nurses talking loudly and laughing. *Noisy nurses.* I turned up the television to drown out the sounds and pulled the covers up to my chin. I wanted the bed that had initially seemed so wonderful to swallow me so I could fade away.

The following day, the albumin and Lasix combination started to work. I got up continuously to use the bathroom. Best feeling ever! Pee! Before my kidney problems, I didn't realize that the everyday process of urinating is magical. Isn't it incredible the basic things we take for granted until they disappear?

Mom left that afternoon, and I took in some *Oprah*, some celebrity news, some snoozing, and some phone calls. Dad visited me that evening after work and brought magazines. "You look different, Jenny. How's it going?" he asked.

"It's working!" My mood pumped up as my weight went down. Every time I went to the bathroom and lost more fluid, I envisioned the return to my "real" self.

When we said goodbye, Dad gently grabbed the tops of my feet that poked out at the end of the bed. "This is to promote healing," he claimed, squeezing to transmit his best energy through my toes. It became the first of his signature toe-grabbing hospital room departures.

When I arrived at the hospital, I didn't realize how much fluid I'd retained because the increasing water retention disguised my shrinking body. Underneath all that fluid, I'd lost weight from the restricted diet. So, after two days, Dr. Brown discharged me from the hospital, thirty pounds lighter.

Well, now, *that* made a difference. Skinny, yes, but my ankles emerged, my face deflated, and my wrists appeared once again. My body was like a new car, and I wanted to take it out and drive around town. Shiny and new. Without that extra fluid, I remembered how I used to feel, how I *should* feel.

I returned to my old self. I wasn't gone!

12.

Arm Puller

BACK HOME, I SPRINTED UP THE STAIRS WITHOUT dragging those heavy tree-trunk legs along. The immobility that had weighed me down like an internal anchor lifted. Spring had sprung, and I could be a part of it.

With *Love, Medicine, and Miracles* under my belt, I incorporated positive thoughts into my self-talk. Stories of people who refused to give in to their disease, tapped into their mind's healing powers, and defied the odds (and sometimes melted cancers through mental strength) gave me hope. *I can do this*, I thought with steadfast determination. *I can heal. This blast of prednisone is going to kick this illness to the curb so I can resume my life.*

At times my self-talk sounded like a fifties tough guy—*kick you to the curb, don't cha know, oh be gone, by golly.* Colorful pops of imagined healing light comprised the background scenery. The mind-body connection became a vehicle that drove my imagined recovery. I envisioned giving my mom and dad a hugely appreciative hug with a tear-filled thank you for bridging this setback. They'd profess great relief as I moved out with fanfare and glory.

I plastered inspirational posters on the walls of my brain. The belief that my mind could overpower my body was essential to propel my hope-fueled existence.

But sometimes doubt dusted my determination. *I will heal! I will. Right? I think I will?* Although the concept that my attitude could produce miracles empowered me, it also pressured me.

The message was one part hopeful, one part accountable. If my thoughts could heal me and turn this around, did the reverse hold true? Had I created this problem through faulty thinking? What if my mental powers couldn't create a miracle?

These questions replayed when I pondered the why, and the why me, of this out-of-the-blue illness. Was it bad eating habits from college? Was it the late nights with microwave popcorn, ceremoniously dunked, one kernel at a time, in low fat "butter"? (The curious consistency beaded into water droplets.) What about Lisa's and my affinity for ketchup, which, to our discerning palettes, made everything better? Did ketchup cause FSGS?

I typically carried an at-the-ready supply of condiments with me. Friends had known me to whip out a bottle of low-fat salad dressing from my purse. At a sorority dinner dance, when people at our table commented on the lackluster chicken, my stash of Grey Poupon saved the night. Was my quirky relationship with condiments-on-the-go a factor in autoimmunity?

Or was our weekend college drinking to blame? Hindsight and memories alchemized with guilt. Everything I had done before was subject to reinterpretation through the lens of illness. Even the word—*autoimmune*—implies the self as the culprit. I had to do everything I could to turn this around. So I tried to pluck invasive weeds of doubt from my garden of positivity by remaining open to alternative methods of healing.

"I heard about this healer today from a friend at the health club," Mom announced one evening. "She knows a woman with lupus who healed after seeing a man in Minneapolis named Terry."

"Terry may be your guy," Dad said with a twinkle in his eye, showing he thought a visit with a healer might be an adventure.

"Let's find out more," Mom suggested. She looked serious. *Might as well try it.*

It turns out that Terry, the healer, was a chiropractor who

used a system called applied kinesiology. His technique used muscle testing to evaluate body imbalances. I'd never heard of this before.

Mom, Dad, and I went to see this magical Terry together, driving to a building near Loring Park in Minneapolis. Dr. Terry called me back to a patient room and started the diagnosis. He looked like a young Dick Clark, eager, spry, and brandishing a full head of cocoa-brown hair. I questioned his white lab coat; was it a costume to impart credentials?

I hopped on his table, and he analyzed my body systems while pushing down on my outstretched arm. He told me to resist the downward pressure while he tested links to various body systems. If I lost strength in my arm, according to Dr. Terry, it was a blaring sign of imbalance. I tried to keep my arm steady each time he pushed it down, yet there were a few times it collapsed under the pressure. I tried. I really did, but I could not hold it up.

His assistant, Sheila, roundly petite and in her fifties, had short, curler-set, honey-blond hair. She gave a wide-eyed glance to Dr. Terry when my arm descended. He compiled his results. Diagnosis: heavy metal poisoning. The cure included a long list of minerals and supplements, which he conveniently sold right there at his clinic. I felt another hit of skepticism. Was he for real? But Terry and Sheila oozed sincerity, and I could tell they wanted to help me. And that's why I was there. I desperately wanted help.

"I'll run your recommendations by my nephrologist," I said, glancing at the printout he'd handed me. "Thank you so much."

When I sheepishly showed this list to Dr. Brown for his approval, he scrunched up his face and eyed me through those professor-like spectacles. "Who told you to take these?"

Unconvincingly, I said, "An internist?" I thought twice about saying, "A chiropractor/healer who pulled on my arm."

"Don't take these," he said firmly. "These could harm you." He warned that my compromised kidneys did not filter my blood like normal kidneys, and these supplements and minerals might build up to dangerous levels.

I felt embarrassed that I had ventured outside of the medical expertise of Dr. Brown and consulted a healer. Yet my powerful motivation for healing (and Dr. Brown's rejection of the alternative supplements) created an itch I wanted to scratch. What if I had heavy metal poisoning and just passed up the cure?

But I complied with the "rules," and since Dr. Brown was the specialist in kidney care, I allowed him to set them. Between applied kinesiology and traditional nephrology, I put my trust in Dr. Brown's multiple years of medical training and experience.

FSGS is but one of many kidney diseases, and it can show up as a mysterious primary infliction, or as a secondary result from infections, viruses, or drug use. I fell squarely into the unexplained category.

Diabetes and high blood pressure are the common causes of chronic kidney disease (CKD). I didn't have either one. And I didn't fit within the demographic groups that face a higher risk —Black individuals and African Americans, Hispanics, Asians, Pacific Islanders, Native Americans, and anyone over the age of sixty.

Although a family history of kidney disease is also a risk factor, CKD had never affected my family. Nevertheless, CKD found me.

That evening, I sat down with my dad in the family room. He sat in his leather chair with a newspaper spread open between his arms. "What did you find out from Dr. Brown?" he asked as he lowered the paper. He seemed curious about how my arm pulling session played to a medical doctor.

"He put the kibosh on the minerals and supplements," I said, and shrugged my shoulders. "I'm really disappointed. I wanted those supplements to work."

"Good thing you checked. You don't want to do any harm by trying to do good."

"I know, but it's frustrating. I don't want to miss out on something that could make a difference."

Dad nodded with understanding. "Let's see what happens at your next appointment." He winked. Acting on a strong recommendation by Dr. Terry, the arm puller, I was about to dip my toe into another unfamiliar specialty.

13.

Music Man

NEXT STOP: MUSICOLOGY. I'D NEVER CONSIDERED THE healing powers of music, but I had nothing to lose. So the following week, Mom, Aunt Lucy, and I drove to an experimental appointment. Seven years separated my mom and her older sister, and their difficult childhoods forged them into a team.

When Mom was five and Lucy was twelve, their father, the grandfather I never met, died from cancer. Widowhood devastated their mom, my grandmother Dodie, a woman in her forties at the time. Dodie immediately sent both sisters to camp for a month and darted off to New York. Lucy resentfully adopted the caretaker role for her younger sister, Liz. But in the years leading to adulthood, their sisterly bond welded into an unbreakable seal.

When the three of us walked into the office, I saw a tall man in his midfifties with a shiny, bald head. His smile flashed large, straight teeth, and he greeted me warmly. Dressed in a short-sleeve button-down shirt tucked neatly into khaki trousers, he looked like a misplaced engineer.

Leading me to a dark room, he genially explained that he'd ask questions while subtle music played in the background. My job was to answer with whatever came to my mind. It sounded easy. And how would this help my kidney function? No clue. But I was game.

Then, and this is a bit of a kicker, he blindfolded me. As one usually is when blindfolded by a musicologist (baffled, uneasy), I suddenly wondered what in the world I had gotten myself into.

He asked questions. I rambled while he played music with varied tempos and tones based on my responses. It sounded nondescript, like Muzak you'd hear while on hold. I recall little about the beginning of the session, but I remember the end. I saw myself in a field with Steve, and we were young.

Sounding like a vulnerable child, I told the musicologist that I didn't like when my brother acted mean (like that time he threw a phone at my head). He suggested I tell Steve. *Well, Steve isn't here*, I wanted to say, but I got the point and imagined doing so. Then he suggested I hit a punching bag. I'm sure it looked like a strange sight—me in the dark with Mr. Music as I tried to whack the bag while blindfolded. Was I supposed to be clobbering Steve? I gave that bag my best shots. (I was still pretty pissed from when he threw my doll Peggy overboard.)

Done. Next?

Then I saw myself approaching a lake. It glistened blue and clear and invited me to jump in. I told Mr. Music I hesitated to jump into the water. He encouraged me to take the plunge. Instead, I cried. My afraid-of-the-imaginary-lake tears sprung from a sensation that an impenetrable wall held me back. The lake looked inviting, downright refreshing, really, and I wanted to immerse myself within it—but something prevented me from leaping into this make-believe water.

"Why can't you jump in the lake?" he asked.

"I don't know," I said as my blindfold absorbed my tears. It became even more awkward as the now-soggy fabric pressed against my face, and I put my hands over my covered eyes. "I really don't know." My tears created a lake of their own.

He told me water frequently represents risk-taking. Maybe the lake represented the life I wanted to jump into, the place I could see in my mind but I couldn't be a part of. Perhaps the water represented the Pacific Northwest, from a recent time that seemed so long ago.

We finished the session. "Can I give you a hug?" he asked before I headed for the lobby.

I hesitated. But I had experienced his support and compassion, so he didn't seem creepy. I said yes. He hugged me long and tight. He wanted me to get better, so I soaked up the energy from my new friend with a unique specialty.

Mom and Aunt Lucy waited for me in the lobby. "Well?" Mom said with raised eyebrows.

"What in the world happened in there?" Aunt Lucy asked, cutting to the chase.

"It wasn't bad. I punched Steve and dealt with some sadness regarding a lake."

"Huh?" Mom said.

"It's hard to explain, but there was music, a blindfold, and some crying and blabbing. Yeah, it was cool. And then he gave me a hug, and I left."

"How inappropriate that he hugged you!" blasted Aunt Lucy, who had recently earned her degree in psychology. "That was a complete boundary violation!"

"Really? Blindfolds, imaginary lakes and punching bags—and you zero in on that damn hug?"

"Boundaries!" she said, laughing with a restrained smile.

"We'll have to file a report with the American Musicology Association, unless, just maybe, they don't have the same rigorous standards as psychologists." I joined her in laughter.

Despite the arm puller and blindfolding musicologist, in time the water weight that I'd lost in the hospital slowly returned. The removal of fluid had been a visual improvement. But it didn't stop the cellular destruction of my kidney cells—amping up the proteinuria and pulling me farther down into the dungeon of the disease. I didn't want to lose that sense of renewal.

Instead, I wanted to be tough and halt my worries with Dale Carnegie-ness. But with each pound of fluid I regained, I focused on my body swelling, my spirits sinking, and my positivity waning. If I could measure my energy as a percentage on a cell phone, I had a low battery warning. Of course I wanted to charge it with a mental miracle, but I had absolutely no control over the events happening to me.

And it was about to get worse.

14.

Face It

"YOU'VE GOT TO TELL LISA," MOM SAID GENTLY. "I don't think she should hold your spot anymore." She knew it was the concession I didn't want to make. Once I told Lisa I couldn't return to our apartment, I would cross the dreaded threshold from temporary to tragic.

Defeated, I retreated to my room. I had visualized returning to the Seattle apartment so intently, and spring was underway. This wasn't the scenario I'd imagined. And now I couldn't see the way out. What was happening to me? I fell into a hard, snotty, ugly, guttural, soul-shaking, deep, rocking, messy, full-force gusher.

I sat on the carpeted floor with my back against the side of my bed. When I finally stopped crying, I called Lisa and told her it wasn't going well. I paused, reluctant to continue. "I *really* didn't want to make this call, Lis, but . . . I can't come back now. I'm in deep here. So, it's time—you should find another room-mate."

Silence. The space between my statement and her response stabbed like a dagger.

"Oh, no. Oh, no. I can't believe it. Are you sure? Isn't the prednisone working?" Lisa's voice came out fast. Urgent.

"No." My voice broke.

"Oh, Jen, I'm so sorry. This is not how it's supposed to go!"

"I know. But you need to move on, okay? Do you have any

potentials?" I asked, and smeared a tear with the back of my hand.

"Well, Denise is looking for an apartment, so I'll let her know."

"Okay. That's good. I'll be back at some point, just not for a while," I said, trying to carve out a future vacancy for me in the universe as a normal person. We planned to have my stuff boxed and shipped.

I hung up and resumed production in the tear factory. That was it, I thought. Denise, Lisa's best friend from high school, would move into our apartment. Life in Seattle would go on. Denise and Lisa would go out for cappuccinos, bring home grocery store sushi, and have late-night conversations while lounging in sweats on the sofa.

I felt I'd begun the divorce process from my rightful place in the world. Looking around, my old childhood room caved in on me. I felt nostalgia for when this room and loving home provided shelter. I had carried a false shield of protection as I set off into adulthood. The shield shattered. My body tensed and my mind raced.

This was the opposite of independence—relying on my parents for financial and emotional support. Not only did the indignity that I'd retreated into parental dependence at twenty-three years old berate me, but also I couldn't even depend on my physical body. Everything seemed to be failing. I wanted to take a super-long nap and give it all a rest.

Later, I came downstairs and curled up on the family room sofa. Mom offered me hot tea and a blanket. Then she sat quietly with me in the silence of my grief.

"What if I'm always going to be alone?" I asked.

"You won't allow it. You'll always be with people—it's your way," she said. "I'm sure of it." But what if she was wrong?

Although Mom eased my emotional state, my physical problems were beyond reach. The water weight kept coming, and with each fluid-saturated pound that accumulated in my cells and on the scale, my desire to be in the world diminished.

That weekend, I borrowed my dad's car and drove around three connected lakes that flank the city of Minneapolis. I sat still and felt stuck as the four wheels turned. Blasting the ethereal sounds of the British band Roxy Music, I emoted to "More Than This," a song that Lisa and I had often cranked in our apartment.

I stared with envy at the lively people—biking, running, walking dogs, talking, laughing, hanging with friends, enjoying ideal lives—a Pepsi commercial beyond my reach. Blue sky. Grass sprouting green. Life in bloom. My hand touched the window that separated me from these "normal" people who seemed to have it all. They were right there . . . so close, yet inaccessible beyond the glass. I sang loudly off-key and pounded on the steering wheel. *Please, prednisone, do your job.*

The trifecta of lousy kidneys, the attack of medication, and my despair created a steady stream of horrible days. Dr. Brown put me back in the hospital. As I packed up the regulars—toothbrush, hairbrush, lotion, underwear, books, notebooks, pens—I considered packing a permanent hospital bag for such occasions. For convenience, like a girl with a prepacked boyfriend bag to make it easy to dash off and spend the night. Except the boyfriend scenario sounded way better.

"You ready?" Mom asked as I walked into the kitchen with my "overnight" bag.

"Yeah. Oh . . . wait, I forgot eyeliner," I said, and pivoted to go back upstairs.

"Eyeliner, really?"

"It's a natural shade of brown. It makes me look less sick," I explained with a sheepish smile.

Mom smiled too, shrugged her shoulders, and said, "Go get it." She was not one to discount the importance of trivial consolations. If a light touch of eyeliner could make anything a wee bit more bearable—well, bring on the eyeliner. *Hospital, here we come.*

15.

Shout Out

THE SAME ROUTINE AS BEFORE—CHECK IN AT THE reception desk, pull out my insurance card, fill out forms. On previous visits, I'd skipped checking a box to declare my religious affiliation, or lack thereof. This time my pencil lingered before I apprehensively checked Catholic, despite my lack of connection to the church.

My parents were raised Catholic and attended Catholic schools. My dad's experience in the church was a confusing medley—a fondness for church traditions mixed with painful memories of harsh treatment (including a nun who tossed him down a flight of stairs a few times as a young boy). Old bruises colored his affinity for traditional worship. That probably explains why Steve and I were raised pseudo-Catholic. (If Catholicism was Coke, we were the Diet Coke version.)

At the progressive church we'd attended as a family, a lively group of crooners pumped up the music—electric guitars, a full drum set, a piano, and a rocking recorder. (No joke, most people think of a recorder as a starter instrument, but this woman really got into it.) We sang Bob Dylan's "Blowin' in the Wind," the Beatles' "Let It Be," and Stevie Wonder's "You Are the Sunshine of My Life."

Yet my die-hard Catholic friends (like Beth and Sheila, with their Irish dad from County Cork) shared hymnbooks, Bible-based sermons, fish on Friday, confessions, and relationships with nuns and priests. I knew none of that. My religious education was minimal. So checking the Catholic box gave me a legitimate reason for pause.

Oh, why not, I decided, *better to belong than to be blank,* so check it I did. Admission complete, Mom and I rode the elevator to the sixth floor.

I walked into the unit and greeted the nurses at the circular central desk. Friendly faces welcomed us back. But as soon as I set my bag down in the room, my identity became bed 22-A. Right from the get-go, I heard a nurse outside the room say, "We need vitals for 22-A."

Similarly, my roommate became just 22-B to me. Here we were, two people sharing space during tough times with minimal connection. The polyester curtain between us divided our illnesses and our lives. When our respective doctors and nurses came to check on us, they would slide the curtain a little farther. It felt like we were zoo animals in separate cages.

This fabric divider blocked sight but not sound. And soundproofing would have been nice. My roommate's voice projected as if through a bullhorn, and she had some very personal circumstances that my mom and I became privy to through proximity. She shouted on the phone about her family issues involving meth addiction, extramarital affairs, drunken brawls, and prison.

Mom and I were a captive audience; we could not turn down the volume or change the channel. An episode of *The Jerry Springer Show* unfolded seven feet away. Shamefully, as if we were audience members, my mom and I listened intently while our mouths gaped open. My head spun on the carousel of her issues. And to think my roommate endured this hospitalization on top of all that! I felt petty that her explosive voice agitated me. But it did. Mom cranked the television's volume and dispensed ice chips for me in a cup.

The unusual events continued. Later that afternoon, a buttoned-up guy with oversized 1970s-style brown glasses walked into my room and stood a few feet from the threshold. He stared straight ahead, bug-eyed, and said, "Just checking the equipment." He turned stiffly and walked out like a robot.

"Good to see they have the A-team on the equipment check today," Mom snickered.

"I bet he comes from a long line of equipment checkers," I said, and we laughed. The humor seemed curative, like a mini-break from the situation. Later, Mom told me that our funniness halted her avalanche of worry when she sat with me. Our ability to laugh restored us both.

Dad came to visit in the evenings. I made phone calls to friends, read magazines, and fell asleep to the background noise of a droning television. The fluid removal treatments were underway. And I was excited to ditch the puffiness. I wanted to experience my body again, even though I knew the last rush of body restoration was temporary. How long would relief last this time? What if I never had relief? My worries kept me awake, and I flipped and flopped to find a comfortable position.

The next day, my roommate went home, and the room became quiet. Then a priest appeared at the threshold and asked if he could offer me a blessing. *Oh, so that's what happens when you check that box.* I clenched with sudden nervousness. "Yes, please?" I answered with an upward inflection, revealing my hesitancy.

I cowered like a Catholic imposter. But I instantly wanted this man, with his bat-line connection to God, to put a higher power on notice. I needed his help to amplify my healing thoughts. My vulnerability fluttered within, like a caged bird trying to escape. I was needy for a force beyond me. *Hello? Anybody out there?*

"What should we pray for?" he asked in the peaceful way a priest should.

"I want to get better." And immediately, tears spilled from my eyes like a faucet. When I said these words out loud, my burden shifted—a deep underpinning of hope and fear dislodged from inside me. I fell to pieces in front of this man, a kind, nonjudgmental stranger, and my emotional nakedness liberated me. It had nothing to do with positivity or visualizations and everything to do with allowing myself to express sad and fearful emotions. And the priest seemed quite comfortable with the puddle of a person I became before his eyes.

He placed his hand on mine, eyes closed, and stated with a gentle intent that we pray for good health. Some traditional crossing followed. A joint recitation of the Our Father.

He left me with tranquility and unleashed something—a gut sense that I was attached to a universal consciousness bigger than me. My feeling didn't fit within a precise dogma, but he stirred my soul. *Does faith have to be neatly packaged? Can it be messy and stuffed away until a crisis comes calling? Is that cheating?* I wondered.

But I knew that this lovely religious man helped me float beyond the confines of my damaged vessel. And I tapped into an enormous energy field of hope. It was freeing. Like a long exhale after holding your breath. In *Creative Visualization*, Shakti Gawain suggests we're all part of the energy of the universe. I wanted that to be true. And at this moment, I believed it was.

And if so, maybe all the people who loved me, and all the people who offered to pray, all the authors who wrote books about healing, all the doctors who devoted years to medical training, all the nurses, musicologists, arm pullers, and now this priest, comprised this universal goodness. It made me wonder, *Is this grand source of collective goodness God?* The idea overwhelmed, covered, and distilled me to my essence. Vulnerable. Seeking. Hopeful.

I opened to a spiritual craving and curiosity. I became small and simple, and everything outside of me expanded. At the same time, my insides felt united with the external world. *And so, if we are all connected, doesn't that mean I belong here?*

16.

Drowning

THE DAYS TICKED BY IN THE HOSPITAL, ON THE SIXTH floor, bed A, room 22. A pseudo-schedule propelled me through the day—as if I were a busy executive with a series of appointments. It started with lab work, a light breakfast, and an awkward, unsatisfying shower.

Time for the housekeeper (well, nurse) to change my linens. A short walk around the floor with my IV pole in tow. Settle in for some local talk show. What's this—lunch, already? More walks, phone calls to friends, a visit with my mom, read, nap, almost time for *Oprah*, then the evening news.

Oh, where has the day gone? It's dinnertime. (Room service . . . so lovely.) Doctors and nurses pop in to interrupt the busy schedule. Visitors come and go. Mom. Dad. Steve. Cousins. Aunts. Uncles. A smattering of friends. News. Primetime. David Letterman . . . and a few unintentionally hilarious infomercials round out the day. Over. And over. And over.

A parade of hospitalists and rounding nephrologists waltzed in with varied medical opinions about the prognosis of my kidneys. Mom and I learned how important it is to have a second set of ears, support, and a notetaker amid a medical circus. She was my advocate. Or, as we affectionately coined her, my "Avocado."

Treatments to remove the extra fluid continued. As the swelling flushed away, my bony chicken legs revealed themselves. As promised, the prednisone stole my muscles. More treatments to go. I stared at the clock. At the television. At my shrinking self. Time seemed as thick as sludge.

I also shared encounters with an eager-to-learn medical team. To be clear, I was not on the enthusiastic side of this equation. As I was buried in my bed, doing my time, a young Doogie Howser ran into the room without introduction.

"Do your legs hurt?" he inquired with an odd level of exhilaration.

"They're swollen, but they don't hurt while I'm in bed," I answered.

"You can get clots! You can get clots in your legs when you don't move. If you have pain, you might have clots!"

"I'm happy you applied your valuable and newly gained clot knowledge to my situation, buddy. Now, please, get out of here." Well . . . maybe I just *wanted* to say that. Good thing he didn't stay long. And oh, how I missed taking a regular shower! It took skill to stand in the tiny bathroom and dodge the plastic curtain's attempt to suction itself onto me. The challenge was significant when paired with IV tubes and rolling metal poles.

Restrictive food and fluid-controlled food trays came and went at mealtimes. One night, a woman from food service raced in with a brimming bowl of peppermints. "I can't get your calories up with all the food restrictions," she said frantically. "Eat these!" A peppermint party. How crazy fun is that?

It was boring stuff.

Until it wasn't.

I woke up suddenly one morning, panic-stricken. *I can't breathe.* My heart pounded. Gasping for air, I fumbled clumsily to hit the call button on the bedside rail.

"Can I help you?" a monotone voice replied through the speaker.

I sat up and thumped my hand on my chest. "Can't breathe,"

I eked. A boa constrictor squeezed my airways, tighter, tighter. Rushing nurses flew into the room. *What's wrong with me? Why can't I breathe!*

"She might have a blood clot or a collapsed lung," one nurse said to another. They were talking over me. It seemed like a dramatic episode of today's *Grey's Anatomy*, but this was no show. I felt overwhelming panic. The frenzy was a blur, and I couldn't speak. The nurses paged Dr. Brown. Additional doctors and nurses swirled frantically around me. Something was terribly wrong. *Is this a code blue? Someone! Help me breathe!* Something blocked my attempts to get air, which made every muscle in my body tighten around my frame like a vise.

Emergency technicians swooped in and took an X-ray in the room. Everyone moved quickly. *Save me.* The film showed abnormalities, and lung specialists filed in to assess the situation. *Please help me get air. Air! I need air!*

Dad walked in, cappuccino in hand, expecting a typical morning visit. His eyes expanded when he saw the scene. Nurses stood on each side of me and held my hands. Eight people crowded into the small room. Dr. Brown rushed in. Dad stood against the back wall. His mouth hung open, and he looked uncharacteristically powerless.

"She has extra fluid in her lungs," Dr. Brown said. "Stop the albumin and increase the Lasix."

Literally and figuratively, I was drowning in myself: drowning in the trapped fluid in my lungs, drowning in my existence, drowning in this disease that pulled me into the water and refused to let go. I struggled to come to the surface.

"We'll take care of this, Jennifer," Dr. Brown reassured me, placing his hand on my shoulder. *Thank God I trust this man.* I closed my eyes. *Please, please, help me breathe. Help me live. Don't let me die.*

Dr. Brown explained my kidneys could not eliminate the water quickly enough, so my fluid-filled lungs struggled to get oxygen. But the nurses executed Dr. Brown's directions, and shortly thereafter my kidneys responded and rid my body of the overloaded fluid. When my lungs cleared, the relief was immediate. Dr. Brown had focused like a skilled pilot with nerves of steel and brought the plane in for a safe landing. Yet even now, I still take extra deep breaths when I remember this crisis.

"Are you feeling a little better?" Dad asked, looking shell-shocked.

"That was bad, Dad. That was so bad." I closed my eyes again. Even though I could breathe now, I felt as solid as a feather in a wind gust. *What if this disease blows me away?*

17.

Independence

THE PREDNISONE MADE MY VEINS SMALL AND UNCOOPERATIVE for the frequent lab draws. Hot packs. Tapping. The lab technicians tried all their tricks. Once, twice, three times . . . no luck. It's all fun and games until your veins don't cooperate.

"You're a tough draw, Jennifer. Next time I'll call the anesthesia department," a frustrated woman said after she failed to get her needle in my vein. That evening, another lab technician gave it a try. He had a pleasant face, sandy hair, and an air of confidence that put me at ease. I hoped he excelled at his job.

I looked away as he approached me with his sharp metal poker. He also struggled to get the needle placed. My body and chest tightened. I held my breath. *Please let this work.*

He whittled. I kept my head turned. He continued to whittle. *What is he doing? This isn't a wood-carving project; it shouldn't take this long!*

I lost it, and huge teardrops streamed down my cheeks. *Is this a CIA torture technique?* He finally finished the job.

"Okay, I got it," he said, sounding relieved.

"Good," I squeaked while looking down to avoid eye contact. I fell into the midst of a mini-breakdown. He gathered up the tourniquet, threw away the alcohol pad and wrapper, labeled the blood tubes, and left the room.

Later that evening, that lab technician popped his head in the door. "Jennifer?" he said timidly. "Sorry to bother you. I'm the guy who made you cry earlier, and I wanted you to know I'm really sorry about that."

"That's okay. I'm fine," I stammered. "It's all of it, not just you. I mean, yeah, no, it's okay. Thanks," I said, flushed with embarrassment, and forced a downcast smile. He smiled and popped back out into the hospital halls. His apology allowed me to realize that we were two regular people. And like my encounter with the priest, when I let unfiltered emotions fly with this considerate stranger, he didn't dismiss me as weak. What do you know? The world didn't stop revolving if my veneer of strength and positivity slipped. Yet this particular lesson was hard to incorporate, so it would circle back again.

What began as a three-day hospital stay stretched into a month. I felt determined to get out of there. During his Friday morning rounds, Dr. Brown said he would observe my fluids over the weekend, check my lab work on Monday morning, and likely discharge me. *Just one more weekend, I can do that!*

After he stepped out, my nurse, Shelly, wrote her name on the whiteboard and ripped the previous day off the little mounted calendar. Another day tossed. Two to go. "I'll set up my own meds this morning," I said.

"I can do it for you, Jennifer," she replied with a boost of peppiness. Her workday had just started, and she looked fresh. I crumpled up in the bed where I'd hung out for thirty days. If there was a contest for buoyant energy between the two of us, she'd win.

"No, thanks. I like to do it myself."

"How about ice chips? And I can help you get up and take a shower," she offered.

"I've got it. Some towels would be great, but I can take a shower myself. Thanks, Shelly."

"You're so independent," she said. "You make my job so easy."

How drastically the markers of independence had changed. Kudos to me. I took my own meds, hobbled down the hall to dispense ice chips in a Styrofoam cup, and stepped into the tiny shower without assistance. Grasping at independence wherever I might find it.

On Monday morning, I woke with anticipation. I was eager to spring from my hospital prison. Bright and early, Shelly handed me a printout of my labs. "Your numbers are worse today," she said.

I grabbed the paper and looked at my results. My creatinine was up. My heart sank. I punched the button that lowered the head of the bed and pulled up the covers. I wanted to disappear under those stiff hospital blankets in protest.

Even when Dr. Brown came into my room, I didn't want to sit up. But I couldn't execute that mini-rebellion because it seemed considerably uncouth to remain flat as he talked to me. And it wasn't like *he* was responsible for the betrayal of my body.

"I'm worried you're not stable," he said tenderly. He knew how much I wanted to get out of there. "I think we need to observe you longer."

These were the words I feared most. No discharge. I squirmed in that godforsaken bed. At first, it had seemed like adjustable comfort heaven; now it was hellish and suffocating.

Dr. Brown said I needed more treatments. The water weight didn't flush off as quickly because my kidney function continued to decline. Was I going to live my whole life in the hospital? Dr. Brown appeared puzzled, and with traces of sorrow on his face, he candidly said, "It's *never* a good thing to be such a fascinating patient."

I got up and pushed my IV pole into the tiny bathroom. Standing there in front of the sink, I turned on the water and started my own waterworks. The only privacy I mustered occurred in this bathroom. The running water helped drown out the sounds of my wails and gulps. It all exhausted me: the repulsive smells of antiseptic cleanser and Betadine, the monotonous background drone of television, medical conversations, beeping machines—the giant hospital hole I could not climb out of.

At night I repeatedly listened to the song "Coming Around Again" by Carly Simon, and focused on the lyrics. *Who's going to come around again? This girl!* Looking back, I blame prednisone-induced insanity (and a glut of hospital time) for the reason I wallowed in song lyrics as if they could set my course.

At the end of the song, a chorus of children sing the nursery rhyme, "The itsy-bitsy spider climbed up the waterspout, down came the rain and washed the spider out, out came the sun and dried up all the rain, and the itsy-bitsy spider climbed up the spout again."

I thought of my mom singing this itsy-bitsy song to me when I was little. Her fingers motioned as the climbing spider and the rain, her arms lifted to illustrate the rising sun, and then her fingers climbed upward again. I wanted to be that climbing spider; I wanted to be that little girl and return to a safe harbor. Would I ever come around again?

18

Better and Bad

DR. BROWN PERFORMED ANOTHER BIOPSY, AND THE results confirmed further progression of kidney damage. My kidneys were not healing. They were failing. I was failing. So Dr. Brown consulted with a team of nephrologists to see if they could use other experimental medications as a last-ditch attempt to reverse the course. They flung the names of potent chemotherapy drugs around, and different doctors had different opinions on whether I should try them.

"You're a young woman," Dr. Brown said as my parents stood by my bed. "Some medications being considered might make you sterile." He lobbed this out as he had with many other side effects, and I didn't register this concept. Not really. Children were not top of my mind at this moment.

I only considered the situation at hand. Being in the middle of a tornado, sterility flew by like another piece of debris. But my dad looked stricken when Dr. Brown tossed that word out. His eyes quickly locked onto my mom's, held her glance, and then stared down at the floor. Mom's eyes filled, and the sadness in the air rose instantly, like a hazy fog.

My mom never questioned if she wanted to be a mother. She'd always loved children, so her decision to be an elementary school teacher was an easy one. When she met and married my dad, they planned to have a family right away. Mom's natural affinity for maternal matters, however, didn't come by way of example. Her glamorous mom, my eccentric grandmother Dodie, leaned more toward self-interest than child-focus. My mom was the baby in her family (with three older siblings). Her oldest brother was sixteen years her senior. And Dodie didn't hesitate to shuffle responsibility for baby Elizabeth onto the older kids. Although many moms repeat the patterns they've seen, my mom was not one of them.

After considerable discussion with the other nephrologists, Dr. Brown said, "We don't know if these drugs will work, and I don't recommend you take them."

Later, I understood my parents' sorrowful reaction to the possibility that their twenty-three-year-old daughter might never conceive children. They realized this blast of illness could eliminate future possibilities at rapid speed. But I didn't know then how the pull of motherhood would grip me later. I couldn't conceive of the future.

"It looks like you're headed toward dialysis, Jennifer," Dr. Brown said glumly, right before he discharged me. I had doubled down on all my creative visualizations to get better. So his words, coupled with the misery I hauled inside my body—the pressure, the fluid, the weakness—crushed me.

I realized my brain had created two compartments: better and bad. I focused mostly on better. *Get better. Get better. Get better.* The bad category existed as a parking lot to store my disastrous notions and deepest fears. I would sort through these thoughts later, only if I needed to. Later came too soon.

We wanted to feel we'd done everything possible, so with Dr. Brown's blessing, my parents and I sought a final verdict from the Mayo Clinic in southern Minnesota. Celebrities and royalty have flocked to this esteemed institution seeking help, so why not me? Off to Rochester we went—the mecca of second opinions and desperation mixed with hope.

We arrived the night before my appointments and stayed at the nearby Kahler Hotel. I'd become a shell of my former self. I dressed slowly and positioned a scarf over my head to hide my lacking locks. My prednisone-wasted muscles made it difficult to walk, and my arms couldn't beat a toddler in a wrestling match. I was a bloated waif.

A skyway connects the hotel to the clinic, so my dad pushed me in a wheelchair while my mom walked by my side. We approached a big circular desk in the middle of an enormous lobby. The seated receptionist looked preoccupied and slightly bored. She handed over a list of tests, labs, and appointments.

I took the schedule and realized this woman provided handouts to ill people day after day. What kind of job was this —working at the sick factory? Patients like me came with hope for their life. She came for a paycheck. How differently we experienced this same space. The contrast unsettled me.

Doling out medical to-dos, she resided safely on the healthy side. I'd crossed the line to the wrong side of life.

After a full day of various procedures, they scheduled me to see Dr. Donaldson, the nephrologist. I hoped he would identify something Dr. Brown had missed. Was I crazy to want him to be a wizard, wave a magic wand, and abracadabra, restore my normal life?

Mom, Dad, and I sat on a long built-in couch in his office and waited. He waltzed in, a fit man in his midfifties with distinguished silver-gray hair and a confident expression. He was a cross between Frank Sinatra and Marcus Welby. "Hello. You must be Jennifer and family," he said.

"Hi, I'm Jennifer," I said unnecessarily. Obviously, I was the patient.

My dad stood to shake his hand. "Hello, Doctor." Something about my dad's face killed me at that moment. He looked so hopeful. My mom sat still in her seat, as if a spinning plate balanced on her head and required considerable focus. It was agony. We were waiting to hear if the promise of my future would evaporate. If only I could stop being a troublemaker. What a complete reversal. This was relegation to a far worse fate than Mrs. Sawyer's corner.

Dr. Donaldson started with friendly banter—I suppose his put-us-at-ease repartee was to establish a buffer of bedside manner. He traded pleasantries with Dad. Mom didn't partake. Although I appreciated the approach, I was not up for the effort.

He looked at my reports and said, "Jennifer, you are a very sick girl. Your kidneys are damaged, and they cannot be repaired. You will need to go on dialysis and have a kidney transplant."

He fired the diagnosis like a cannonball. I sucked in a quick breath and hunched forward. His words ripped into me. I wanted to escape this room, this clinic, and my body. I felt like giving up right then and there.

My parents' eyes dropped. I had let them down. How could I have done this to them? How could my body have done this to me?

Dr. Donaldson was not done. "Jennifer, you probably feel horrible right now. Your body is filled with toxic side effects from prednisone."

I sat motionless and stared at Dr. Donaldson. "You will get off this medication and become stronger," he continued. "Your hair will grow back, and you'll feel better when you're on dialysis. This is the worst of it. You're on your way to feeling better."

I clung to his words. *This is the worst of it. You're on your way to feeling better.*

As we stepped out his office door, he spotted the wheelchair parked a little ways down the hall. "You know, I've seen people so weakened from medications they arrived at my office in a wheelchair. Good luck to you," he said, and offered a sympathetic pat on the shoulder.

My mom and dad and I looked at each other, our mouths slightly agape, and waited for him to retreat into his office and close the door.

"He seemed like a bright guy, but he was pretty dim-witted about that wheelchair situation," Dad said.

"Quick, get me out of here before he sees it's mine," I said in a rush, as if we were about to commit a grand theft wheelchair crime. At that tiny moment, we laughed. The elevator descended to the first floor. Clumped together in the lobby, devastated, we hugged each other. The hope we held on to poured through the sieve of our second opinion.

My dad looked up with wet eyes and choked out, "I think it will all turn out okay." The pilot light of his Dale Carnegie optimism still burned.

My eyes reddened; I tamped down the rush of panic and said in a crackly voice, "It has to." Then we just stood there together in a silent huddle.

On the way home, Dad turned on the radio. Looking out the window from the back seat, I gazed at the blue sky and felt mismatched with the weather. I was incompatible with May. Bob Marley's "Three Little Birds" played from the speakers. The reggae filled the car interior with rhythmic conviction. A sweet song. A melody pure and true. A message. Don't worry about a thing.

"I like this song," my dad said. "I think this guy is right."

"It's a good song, Dad."

"Every little thing is gonna be all right." Mom repeated the lyrics as if she was trying to convince herself. She wiped a cascading tear from her cheek.

I sat back, closed my eyes, and tried to fold those lyrics into my thoughts. Dad bopped his head back and forth to the music, and Mom turned her head toward the window. Bob Marley briefly soothed our souls.

Yet as we drove home together, north via Highway 52, I had absolutely no clue where this road would take me.

19.

A Promise

AT HOME, MOM EXPLAINED THE DOCTOR VISIT OVER A
series of phone calls to friends and family. Her voice sounded
flat, her delivery straightforward, like a news reporter reading
lines without personal inflection. We plodded through the space
that surrounded us, concentrated and thick, as if propelling
through a vat of mud.

I heard Mom explain it to Aunt Lucy. "No, they are sure.
Her kidneys are far too damaged. Yes. Dialysis. Probably soon.
Then transplant. Yes, but I don't know when. She's upset, yes.
I'm hanging in there. Please do tell them. Thanks. I'll keep you
posted." She was softly weeping all the while.

Weeping right along, I went upstairs to my bedroom and
called Lisa. I formed the words I never wanted to: "It didn't
work. My kidneys are failing. Dialysis soon. Transplant eventually." I called Rae. Same words.

I went back downstairs and stood by Mom as she stared
out the open window over the kitchen sink. It didn't seem right
that birds had the nerve to chirp cheerful notes of summer. I
burrowed in for a hug and wanted to collapse into her side and
disappear.

"I can't stop crying," I said. My voice came out in an uneven
warble. How was I supposed to visualize my life now that getting
better was no longer possible? Had love, medicine, miracles, and

obsessive visualizations failed me? Apparently. I didn't have the mental tools to manifest the right outcome, and an avalanche of sorrow crashed over me. The answer to my question arrived. Heal or fail? Fail.

"I can't stop either," Mom said. Her voice shook with the same fragile frequency, and redness rimmed her eyes.

"But what if I really can't stop?" I asked.

"I think we should decide to *not stop*." Her tone strengthened, and she turned to face me. "We're going to cry for the entire day. No stopping allowed. We need to cry—and *that* is what we're going to do. To hell with it."

Mom stood so resolute in this mission; she made me laugh while I cried. What a transformative trick—how did she consistently elicit laughter in the most unfunny of moments?

"Okay then. That's settled," I said. "An all-day cry-fest."

We did different things. I cleaned up some stuff in my room, and Mom paid bills. I threw in the laundry. Mom read. And throughout the entire day, futzing around, tissues in hand, we cried for hours. But Mom said she couldn't eat. "You've got to have something, Mom," I implored. Insisting she sit down, I made her a sandwich.

When I couldn't cry anymore, I went to Walgreens to pick up a prescription. I ambled down an aisle—makeup on one side and nail polish on the other. I passed point-of-purchase displays featuring perfect skin, shiny lips, and smoky eyes. Arriving at the prescription pickup line, I stood behind a row of older people. I may have been the feeblest one among us. How unsettling. It didn't seem age appropriate to recognize myself in these elderly folks. *Hey friends, I shuffle and take meds too! High five! I'm twenty-three!*

Back home, low on energy and spent from the flood of tears, I replayed Dr. Donaldson's promise of better days ahead. I hoped he was right. A kidney transplant didn't sound like a riot to me, but I needed to believe his prediction of a rosier future so I could keep moving forward.

PART TWO

———

WISHING

"Once you choose hope, anything's possible."

—Christopher Reeve

20

See Me

WHEN DR. BROWN EXPLAINED A SURGEON WOULD connect an artery in my left forearm to a vein, it made me cringe. Eventually, this connection would enlarge the vein so it could accommodate obnoxious-sized needles. "You will have an AV fistula to make dialysis possible," he said.

I arrived at the hospital for the surgery, a same-day procedure, and learned I would only receive relaxation juice, not full anesthesia. Bright lights buzzed overhead as I lay flat on a platform in a cold room. A nurse appeared at my side and gave me a light bump of sedation. "You let me know if you feel any pain," she instructed.

The surgeon strutted in with great bravado. He glanced around with beady brown eyes, golden brown hair, tan skin, and the cocky presence of an actor stealing the stage. "Let's get this show on the road," he boomed. "Where's my music?"

Then country music filled the room, and he sang along, loud and proud. I was glad *one* of us was having fun.

"We're going to set you up with a fistula today. Sound good?" he asked.

"Yep." It didn't sound good, but whatever.

Midway through the procedure, I felt an uncomfortable tightness. I grimaced. "What's wrong?" the assisting nurse asked.

"I have some pain."

"Where, Jennifer? Where is the pain?"

"My chest," I said with constricted breath.

"She reports pain in her chest!" the nurse shouted.

"Goddamn it! I may have punctured her lung. Goddamn it! These goddamn nephrotics have shitty veins. Goddamn nephrotic!" the doctor shouted over my outstretched body on the operating table. *Holy shit, what is happening?*

The blood pressure cuff squeezed my arm. The nurse said, "Her blood pressure is really high." Of course it was high—the doctor just shouted that I was a goddamn nephrotic! Is it possible to avoid high blood pressure when the doctor performing your surgical procedure is losing it?

"Just breathe, Jennifer. It could be a stitch, a catch in your side from not breathing deep enough. Just breathe," the nurse said calmly. "In . . ." She took a long breath in as a guide. "Out . . ." She exhaled. I inhaled as she instructed and pushed it slowly back out. The cramped discomfort eventually dissipated, and the pain subsided. No lung punctures.

The lunatic doctor's outburst, however, continued to pierce me. I struggled to regain myself and process what had just happened. I figured I'd probably have permanently high blood pressure now, as an aftershock from the tension I absorbed in that room.

Later, I would see *The Elephant Man* and sympathize with his emotional plea, "I am not an animal! I am not an animal! I am a human being."

I should have bellowed, "I am not a goddamn nephrotic!"

After the procedure, the doctor left, and the nurses removed the surgical cap from my head. The bandana that had covered my mostly gone hair slipped off. I froze with the accidental exposure.

A nurse said, "It's hard to wash your hair in the hospital,

huh?" I saw her shoot a glance at the other nurse. What did that glance mean? Were they laughing at me?

I wanted to scream, *You don't realize this isn't me! I have thick hair, really—well, I used to less than a year ago—and my cheeks were full, and my eyes were shiny like a twenty-something-year-old's eyes should be. I'm a recent college graduate with friends and a soon-to-be career. Don't look at me like I'm an emaciated, thin-haired, bandana-clad girl with a pale face and bony arms and legs. You people think I'm a goddamn nephrotic—but you don't see me!!!*

I got more than I expected during that procedure. My fistula had been placed, but my spirit had been crushed.

21

It Begins

THEY SET MY DIALYSIS SCHEDULE FOR MONDAYS, Wednesdays, and Fridays, 1:00–4:00. Before my first procedure, Mom and I went to the unit for a tour. That's where we met Sue, the social worker. In her midforties, she wore her dark hair in a sleek bob and dressed in a navy A-line skirt with a white blouse. Sue spotted me right away. My attempt to conceal a wig with a scarf tied around my head, or perhaps my general look—a terrified, confused girl without kidney function—gave it away.

With a gentle voice, Sue gestured at the machines like a real estate agent about to present the features of a property listing. Then she introduced us to a strawberry-blond, freckle-faced, muscular man. "Tom is our lead technician."

"Jerry, Anne," she said to the other technicians across the room, "meet Jennifer." Both Jerry and Anne, dressed in blue scrubs and clogs, were tending to the machines and elderly patients. My stomach tightened.

"Hi, Jennifer!" they both greeted me, accidentally in unison, and laughed.

I glanced toward them but didn't want to stare too long at the blood-soaked filters attached to each patient because my gut started to churn and flip.

"We run this place like an AA meeting," Jerry quipped in recognition of the singsong greeting. "Get ready." His face was genial; he looked like a younger J. K. Simmons (*Whiplash* Academy Award winner and the guy in the Farmers Insurance commercials).

"Good to know," I said. I tried to remain calm as Sue continued the tour, but as she explained the process, her words blurred like static. Smacked by facts and fears. *Boom, boom, boom.* Faces closing in, Mom's compassion, Sue's attention, strangers attached via tubes to whirling machines, the eager-to-greet-me technicians.

Everywhere I looked, I saw blood and wrinkled faces.

My rumbling insides rose upward. I felt panic register on my face and looked at Sue. "Bathroom?" She pointed. I ran and made it just in time to throw up in the toilet. Reeling, I splashed water on my face, rinsed out my mouth, and rearranged my scarf. As my heart pounded, I gave myself advice. *Be tough. Pull it together. You can do this.*

The next day, my first treatment began. Stiffly, I sat in a vinyl chair and pulled the side lever that propped up my legs. Tom (the lead technician I'd met the day before) connected all the lines and pushed a bunch of buttons. The pumps started to spin. A cartridge filtered my blood, like a washing machine, to remove the waste. I closed my eyes and listened to the humming machines, nearby patient voices, snores, and the cacophony of televisions. The pervasive smell of plastic and disinfectants gave me a slight headache.

Three hours later, it was done.

One successful treatment down. Tom explained I'd be tired from the shift in my blood chemistries and preached compliance. "Remember your diet and fluid restrictions. It's crucial. Watch the fluid carefully." This was important advice because everything I drank would stay with me until my next treatment. (It's remarkably strange when you no longer pee.) "If you come in next time with too much fluid on board, it makes for a tough run," he said. I didn't know what that'd look like, but I didn't want to find out. I'd been warned. Tom placed his hand on my shoulder. "You've got this, kid."

But did I?

Three days a week, drive to the hospital. Sit down in the waiting room. Wait until a technician claimed me. Step on the massive scale (like the contestants did years later on *The Biggest Loser*) and see how many kilograms I registered over my "dry weight." (Dry weight is what you would weigh if you'd peed.) I balled up my fists with tension before the digital number popped up. The scale was the judge of how well I'd resisted my thirst since my last treatment.

If I drank too much and needed a lot of fluid removed, I risked severe cramps, crashing blood pressure, and passing out. Knowing that menu of trouble, I did my best to restrict the lure of thirst-quenching beverages.

A few treatments later, I sat down and extended the leg-lift lever to put my feet up. Jerry started the machine and offered me cranberry juice. This was my "free" drink because the treatment removed these fluid ounces during the run. Cranberry juice became nirvana. And ice? Don't get me started on how heavenly crushed ice can be when you're in a perpetual state of thirst.

"Hello, Jennifer," Olga, a fellow patient, unleashed her low, gravelly smoker's voice to greet me. Her teased, mousy-gray hair resembled the texture of cotton candy, and the slump of her posture reflected her eight-plus decades of life. She barked to Tom, "Hey, get me two apple juices, would ya?" Then she declared, "Aw, I love you, Tom." She had small, tough veins, but Tom could always successfully place her needles. Although Tom and Olga were complete contrasts—strong versus weak, sharp-minded versus scattered, vital versus on the decline—they shared a sweet technician/patient compatibility.

Tom handed Olga one juice instead of two. "You drank too

much since Monday, Olga. I can't pull that much fluid safely."

She pooh-poohed him with a "humph" and a stern shake of her head. "Oh, Tom . . . you don't understand!" she exclaimed in her distinctive deep voice. (She sounded a smidge like James Earl Jones.) "I watch my programs, and during these commercials, I see all the food and drinks. How in the world do you expect me to be careful when I see all those darn commercials?"

Her words were funny, but I understood. I obsessed over David Letterman's beverages while he interviewed guests. Who does that? A thirsty girl, that's who.

Don't drink. Watch the diet. Don't drink. Watch the diet. Diet. Diet. Diet.

In the summer between ninth and tenth grade, my body plumped up like a soaked raisin. My jeans tightened around my thighs, my tush rounded, and my chest kept popping. And none of it felt comfortable. These changes approached like a tidal wave, so I set out to halt the metamorphosis with willpower, dedication, and dieting.

When I was in high school, as now, diet mania was everywhere. The cabbage soup diet, the Beverly Hills diet, the Scarsdale diet, and the fruit diet. Weight loss articles shouted from every magazine in the grocery store checkout lane. Tab, the diet soda, was for beautiful people. I had focused on my calories with rigid precision. If calories and I were courting, I was the fickle Victorian. *I want you, but no, no, I mustn't. You tempt me, but I will not let you take me.*

When I accidentally grabbed a regular pop from the pantry instead of the zero-calorie variety, an epic crisis ensued. Noticing a lingering, delicious aftertaste, I checked the can. One hundred and twenty calories! A mad panic overcame me, as if I had swallowed poison. This sugar-pop calamity was a clue—when I set my mind to something, in this case, calorie restriction, I could be obsessive and rigid. It didn't serve me well when I locked myself in a calorie-controlled prison.

Severe food restriction to change your body size quickly instigates a fight with your brain. But biology ensures that your brain is a formidable opponent. I cringe now at the thought of teenagers boarding the merry-go-round of diets. It's fraught with complications. Unrealistic beauty ideals cause body dissatisfaction. Body dissatisfaction can lead to dieting. Dieting leads to hunger. Hunger prompts your brain to crave food. Cravings lead to overeating. Overeating leads to body dissatisfaction. And round and round it goes.

Eventually, I abandoned the notion it was admirable to undereat. Freedom. I exercised regularly, substituted healthy choices for diets, and regained a more wholesome and intuitive relationship with food.

But now body dissatisfaction stirred into a different recipe, not of body size but of body betrayal through autoimmunity and crappy kidneys. My teenage foray into controlling food choices with precision circled back around with chronic kidney disease. My ability to exercise control served me well as a compliant devotee of the dialysis diet.

Compliance was critical, but a significant number of kidney patients did not follow the food and fluid restrictions carefully. I'm not surprised. It's difficult. But it's also a very serious undertaking because diet noncompliance can cause significant health issues. Or worse, death.

My foods were no longer measured in calories but in fluid ounces, saltiness, potassium milligrams, and phosphorus counts. I measured my vegetables. I brought food scales to restaurants to weigh my proteins. I eliminated salt from recipes. As I tackled this new brand of diet focus, it might have been mistaken for disordered eating, but that wasn't true at all. Kidney disease flipped my perception of the thinness ideal and dieting culture on its head. Extreme thinness advertised illness. I craved health.

22.

Fun Again

NICK AND I HAD EXCHANGED LETTERS AND SPOKE A FEW times while he lived in London, but so much had happened since I last saw him in Seattle. Most of the time, I wanted to hide from the world, so I was glad he wasn't around to witness my demise. In that respect, his overseas travel worked out well.

But now he was coming to Minnesota to visit, and I felt equal parts excited and terrified. The bummer was I sported a wig and still had a clunky port taped to my skin beneath my collar. On the upside, the prednisone side effects had lessened, reducing my puffball-ness. Dialysis stabilized me, and as promised, I felt better.

I gripped tightly to the steering wheel as I drove to the airport to pick him up. I checked myself in the rearview mirror a thousand times. Far from perfect, I squinted to find any traces of cuteness in my reflection. Compared to when I was at the Mayo Clinic, I looked pretty darn good.

Walking through the crowded airport, I chewed on my lower lip and feared an anxious sweat might overtake me. Then I spotted Nick at a distance through the thick mess of travelers with wheeling bags. His wavy golden hair, sea-blue eyes, and athletic muscular build appeared as I jumped to see over heads. I caught his attention with a raised wave. His smile was enormous, and I wanted to skip.

"Why hello, stranger," he said with that familiar voice, that familiar face, that way of his that seemed oddly nostalgic, being it represented a time and place that existed not so long ago.

My self-consciousness melted away. We hugged and laughed nervously.

"You made it sound like you were Quasimodo, but you look good," he said. "Definitely skinny, cute wig, but you know, good."

"You're a good liar," I replied with immense relief. Then we bubbled into conversation, as always. We couldn't talk fast enough—London adventures, dialysis stories (as if they were equal), funny tidbits of what we had to catch up on.

"Hello, Cramers," Nick said as we walked into the kitchen where Mom and Dad sat enjoying a glass of wine. They'd already met Nick a few times during college visits.

Mom stood to give Nick a hug. "Well, hello. Good to see you."

"Nick!" Dad exclaimed while extending his hand for a firm shake.

"Looks like your daughter has fallen into quite a mess here," Nick said as he put his arm around me. He tried to be light, but it came out like a cheesy used car salesman spewing forced conversation. Mom and Dad rolled with it. We all knew it was a tough circumstance, so everyone deserved some leeway.

"I'll say." Mom looked at me and smiled.

I took Nick upstairs and showed him Steve's room, where he would stay during his indefinite visit. A one-way plane ticket ensured a relaxed and open-ended stay. While he unpacked the contents of his bag neatly in the closet, I sat on the bed.

"It's crazy you're here," I said. "I feel like I've gone through a war since I last saw you." Leaning against the wall while crossing one leg on top of the other, I couldn't wrap my mind around this. We were just in my Seattle apartment. Boom, random kidney disease catapulted me out of there, and here we were sitting in my brother's room in Golden Valley.

"I think you have," he said as he finished placing a stack of polo shirts and folded jeans on shelves. He stepped out of the closet and sat down next to me. "Let's bring some fun back into your life."

"I don't understand . . . what is this 'fun' you speak of?"

"Fun is like riding a bike. You'll remember soon enough." He grinned. I liked the banter and the sentiment. But could I ever experience fun again in the same way?

My mom loved Nick's sense of humor. The two of them created an alternate name game—you just pick whatever new name you desire. Sitting around the kitchen table, my mom chose Vanessa. (Vanessa Redgrave may have inspired her choice.) Nick selected Christopher.

"What about you? What's your new name?" he asked. I rested my hand under my chin and went into deep contemplation.

"Bianca," I replied.

"No, no. That's no good." Nick scrutinized my face.

"It's good. I'm going with Bianca," I said with satisfaction.

Mom chimed in, "No, that doesn't do it."

"Bianca is exotic," Nick said. "You're too wholesome for Bianca."

What was the deal with these two? "Back off, this is my fantasy name," I retorted, with thoughts of being dark and edgy like Bianca Jagger, Mick's first wife. Why not a glamorous jet-setting woman with a rock star husband? Who could be further removed from my medical mayhem in Minneapolis? Wasn't that the point of fantasy?

This random, off-the-wall absurdity was precisely what we needed. Nick's playfulness temporarily pulled me back to when I knew nothing about biopsies or failing kidneys. We went to movies, shopped, and enjoyed the low-key, nondescript hanging out I'd missed. He filled in gaps of loneliness and added a fun balance to the medical activities that had consumed my life. He came along to my medical events as well, pulling up a chair and keeping me company during the hours spent in the dialysis unit.

During a hospital stay, I remember Nick outstretched next to me in the bed. Side by side, we watched television. And I felt so happy. Here we were, together, laughing like we'd done in college. The setting was shitty, but still. The sharp edges of loneliness eased because he was there.

Lisa came to visit that summer too. Lisa, Nick, and me, together again. We ventured off to the state fair, and I pointed to a strap-in ride that suspended your body upside down on a curved loop. Laughing, I said, "Wouldn't it be hilarious if I got on that ride and my wig fell off?"

Lisa smiled gently, but Nick's face fell. "Nobody would laugh if they saw you without a wig. That wouldn't strike anyone as funny." His seriousness hit me. My attempt to be lighthearted didn't land, and his reaction highlighted the heaviness of my reality.

Meanwhile, Mom thought a puppy would be a lovable distraction while I bided my time. I agreed. Who doesn't get uplifted by a puppy? So Mom, Nick, and I drove to a breeder's farm in northern Minnesota and picked out a wheaten terrier pup. We named her Mickey. She inspired our spontaneous bursts of "Oh Mickey, you're so fine, you're so fine you blow my mind. Hey Mickey!" We all giggled during Mickey's random bouts of the zoomies—wild-eyed, spirited sessions where she ran in frenetic circles and then collapsed. Watching all that energy on display boosted mine.

Shortly before Nick arrived, Rachael moved back home. Soon after that, our high school tribe all found their way back to Minneapolis. Liz, Suzanne, Amy, and Carrie. My people were back in town!

On weekends, Nick and I hit up parties at Rachael's house near the University of Minnesota campus. I became socially restored, enjoying the normal activities of a twenty-three-year-old girl with a boyfriend, with just a few limitations: frequent nauseousness from kidney failure and dialysis, especially in the morning; always feeling cold; and fluid restricted.

Denying my thirst wasn't easy. To battle the overpowering temptation to go on ice water binges, I would fill a big glass with ice cubes. It lasted so much longer.

Sour lemon gum and sugar-free candies helped too. Fluid lust overcame me when I watched "regular" people drink beverages. My obsession was inescapable even when I slept. Nightmares of drinking and drinking and drinking, jug after jug of water, populated my resting brain. Then I'd wake up in a panic until the initial grogginess would yield to relief.

Just a nightmare. It's over. You're okay. I daydreamed of feeling that same sense of enormous relief after my transplant.

23

Dim

TREATMENT AFTER TREATMENT, WEEK AFTER WEEK, dialysis became my new routine. "Jennifer Cramer, come on down!" Jerry (the playful technician with a sparkly sense of humor) called my name one afternoon when the chair was ready. Walking toward him, I feigned excitement like a contestant descending the steps on *The Price Is Right*. Dialyzing patients lined each side of the room, and I smiled and greeted my new kidney failure friends.

Olga had become one of my favorite characters at the unit because I never knew what would fly out of her mouth. "Hey," she said to me one afternoon, "you're a cute kid. I hope you don't get murdered."

"Olga . . . what?" Tom said, furrowing his eyebrows. Jerry grinned and shrugged his shoulders. We all laughed. Although Olga was prone to absurd outbursts, she was endearing.

The other twenty-three-year-olds I knew mostly had friends their own age and viewed the world through the same lens. Boring! Or so I tried to spin it. *My* lucky life was also peppered with technicians, doctors, senior citizens, and outburst-prone Olga. But it's true that where I first saw wrinkly faces, now I saw friends. Dialysis eventually became like a treatment version of *Cheers*, the welcoming place to hunker down where everybody knows your name. A silver lining of sorts, and I was in pursuit of the bright side.

"You're young. You be careful, kiddo," Olga said.

"Don't worry, Olga. I'm always on the lookout for murderers," I assured her with a big smile. I felt certain I'd never said *that* before.

Then Nick and I started to have dumb arguments about hypothetical situations. So silly. *If you were super rich, you'd buy this kind of car. No, I wouldn't. Yes, you would!* Obviously, they weren't about what they were about. I sensed Nick's playfulness shift into a denser mood. His sparkle became intermittent, like a flickering light bulb, as the initial adrenaline from our reunion dimmed.

I got tired; Nick got wild. I measured and carefully limited every ounce of fluid. And Nick enjoyed too many ounces of alcohol.

One evening, at one of Rachael's house parties, we absorbed loud music, a bit of beer, and much-needed social energy. As the night continued, Nick's buzz transformed into visible intoxication. When I was ready to go, I couldn't find him. My friend Ned said he'd spotted Nick bolting out the door in a sloppy dash—running full speed into the night.

"Where did he go?" I asked.

"I don't know. He was freaking out," Ned said.

It was late, Nick hadn't returned, and I left. He eventually made his way back to Rae's and bummed a ride home. The following morning, when he came into the kitchen, I asked what'd been going on the night before. I stirred honey into a steaming mug of tea and looked at him for an explanation.

"I had too much to drink. I had to get out of there." He flung open the refrigerator and hunted for something to grab.

"What made you take off like that? Are you okay?" I wasn't sure if I felt responsible, worried, embarrassed, or ticked off. "Is this situation too much?"

"No, don't be crazy. We're good." He shot those words out too fast—a troubled energy radiated from him like an uncomfortable heat.

Where'd the fun go? Is he in trouble? And where in the world is this relationship headed?

24.

Freak

DAYS LATER, A CLEAR, BRIGHT SUMMER SKY SUMMONED.
"Let's go to the lake today," I suggested. Nick was game.

"Great, we'll pack a picnic lunch and hang out at Lake Calhoun." I wanted to be one of the vibrant people of Minneapolis, taking advantage of the signature city lakes. It was an about-face from the previous summer when I depressingly drove my dad's car in lake loops and waited for prednisone to solve all my problems.

I shook the memory and took a deep breath of gratitude. Things were better. I went upstairs to throw on shorts and a T-shirt and stared at my exposed legs. Visible ankle bones made me happy. Wrapping a floral-patterned scarf around my wig, I wiggled my feet into some flip-flops and grabbed towels. Downstairs, I assembled sandwiches and packed a beach bag for our picnic.

"Look at those twiggy bird legs," Nick said.

"I will never take my ankles for granted again," I replied with a big smile.

"To the beach!" He wrapped me in his arms and gave me a tight squeeze. Here he was. I absorbed his glimmer again.

We claimed a spot on the sand with our towels and spread out our lunches. As we plopped down, I enjoyed every ray of sun that heated my skin and baked me into contentment. Like that sense of arrival you feel when slipping into a warm bed after a dog-tired day, I allowed the comforts of this moment to permeate me with happiness.

"Minneapolis is a great city," Nick said right before he chewed a bite of his turkey sandwich. "I could live here."

I considered that his view of the city differed from mine—it was more than just a place to land after illness interrupted life. I looked across the lake. Was that just a simple statement, or did he want to live here? I took it as a passing comment and let it be.

"I miss Seattle. But I agree, Minneapolis is cool, and my parents are so supportive. I don't know how I'd get through all this without them." I stood up to stretch my legs and walked to the shoreline. When I returned, I leaned over to grab a water bottle, and my PICC line (peripherally inserted central catheter) popped out from under the tape that secured it to my chest.

"Conceal that!" Nick said. Startled, I looked down to see the red and blue tabs on the end of the line sticking out. I tucked them back in quickly. "We should go," he insisted. His body tightened as he swiftly shoved our garbage into the paper bag.

"Why? What's wrong?"

"That tube came out. People could see it. I don't want people to look at you like you're a freak." His mouth pulled into a tight straight line on his face.

A brick dropped within me. "People will look at me like I'm a freak?" I paused to take that in. "Forget about 'people.'" I held up my fingers to form air quotes around the word and continued, "People don't matter. What do you think? Do you think I'm a freak?"

"I'm just squeamish about tubes and stuff like that, so I bet other people are too. I want to protect you from people staring at you," he said, standing. He seemed in a hurry.

The last thing in the world I wanted to be was a freak. My eyes burned with tears of shame. I wanted to disappear, but Nick held an unflattering mirror up to my illness, and I hated the reflection. Maybe I didn't belong on this beach after all. How could I have hoped his arrival would bring part of me back?

We weren't having a lovely time reconnecting now. Everything was different. Everything had gone to shit.

"Sorry if I'm protective," he said.

Passive-aggressive protection is not protective. I don't know if I said that out loud or not; it's a blur. I just remember I grabbed the towels and shook them hard to shake everything off and away.

As I walked toward the car, I turned around and took a long look at the people that remained, those unencumbered people living healthy, freak-free, tube-free lives. What would it take to join them again?

25

Reject

I NEEDED GIRLFRIEND ADVICE, PRONTO, SO I CALLED LISA from my bedroom. Nick, Lisa, and I had hung out like the Three Musketeers on campus, so I assumed she'd have some insight. I told her about the lake fiasco and how Nick was drinking.

"What are you going to do?" she asked.

"I don't know—if he's freaking out, he should leave. It's a drag for both of us."

She hesitated for a moment before she said, "Jen, I don't think he knows where to go."

"What do you mean?" I felt an ominous feeling as I rocked back and forth.

"Nick told some guys he wants to be with you because he doesn't have a job lined up in Seattle. He needs the free place to stay." Lisa spoke softly, as if her gentle volume would lessen the blow.

"He needs the free place to stay?" My voice became elevated while my brain exploded. "I've become the free place to stay? What do I even do with that?" I fumed.

"I didn't want to say anything," Lisa continued, "but you don't need that shit right now. Do you want him to stay?"

"I don't know what I want anymore. But thanks for telling me. That's good to know."

"What a dick!" she exclaimed with the satisfying and proper vengeance only a close girlfriend can offer.

I pressed my hands over my ears as if that would contain the sudden free-for-all of cascading thoughts. Ping. *He's an ass.* Ping. *How will you ever be in another relationship?* Ping. *Look at you, living here in your parents' house.* Ping. *Sick girl.* Ping. *Stay positive, you got this.* Ping. *Be tough.* Ping. *Where will this all end for you?* Ping. *Would it be so bad to be alone?*

I covertly talked to my mom about Nick in her bedroom with the door closed. Mom said, "I think he's been drinking in the middle of the day." She'd seen Nick hovering by the sink tucked behind the hinged walnut doors of the family room bar. The glass shelves held spirits, and my parents served drinks there during holidays and parties. When Nick saw her, he pushed back a bottle of vodka and dashed away with an ice-clinking glass.

"Really?" I asked, surprised. Concerned. "He drinks at parties, but in the middle of the day? He's struggling more than I thought."

We both raised our eyebrows in unison and shared an oh-no look. "What are you going to do?"

"I don't know, Mom, but it isn't looking good."

Nick stopped coming with me to my treatments. And his reaction on the beach, as though I had leprosy, drilled me further into a spiral of loneliness. I contemplated my future romantic life. If any. My once lofty twenty-two-year-old notions of promise were snuffed out like fingers to a candle flame.

The next day, I sat with Nick in the family room on the sofa and asked him about the drinking. I tried to be kind, but I'm sure anger and sadness saturated my tone. He denied it. His eyes darted around the room while his arms folded inward like a collapsible cardboard box. He said nothing; he didn't have to—his body language told me everything. He wasn't in a good place.

I asked him how he felt about the rest of it. The health stuff. "Is this too much for you?" The question made me want to burst into tears, so my lower lip did a little dance.

He admitted he didn't want to go to dialysis with me anymore because it made him uneasy. "You know I hate hospitals. It makes me feel like I'm going to get sick. I'm so uncomfortable there," he explained.

"Yeah, I get it. It's pretty uncomfortable for you," I said, brimming with sarcasm. Who likes hospitals? That's like a father-to-be bemoaning his exhaustion as he watches his wife undergo childbirth. What a wimp. But the childbirth analogy had a fatal flaw. Because this was not his kid, or in this case, kidney. He couldn't handle it, and he didn't have to.

"Don't go anymore," I said, resigned to the reality that this was not working. How nice would it be to say that I didn't want to show up there anymore? I'd like that too. If only it were a choice for me. Resentments rose.

I'd become unmoored—nothing about our current time and place resembled our Seattle lives. Nothing about me resembled my previous self. Nick was struggling. I was struggling. The combination was too much. I needed to focus my energy on my health, and I knew he needed an environment more supportive than I could provide.

"You need to go," I said. Steady voice. Arms crossed.

He begged me to let him stay because he claimed he couldn't afford to live anywhere else. Here was a person I'd cared about for so long, pleading with me. My emotions unsteadied me, but I resisted. "That's an insufficient reason. Just figure something out."

"Please, I'll be better. It's just hard. I know I'm horrible. But you're horrible too. This isn't easy," he said. *Was I horrible too?* "Like you always say, everything always works out in the end." He sounded desperate, but I didn't want him around anymore, with his mean comments and his excessive fluid consumption. Come on. And to think he used to love me.

"I was wrong, Nick. Everything does *not* always work out in the end." He sunk further into the couch, and I walked away to preserve my resolve. It was quiet when he placed those neatly folded polo shirts back in his suitcase. When I dropped him off at the airport, he hugged me, and we said goodbye. Tears streamed down my face on the drive home. Summer had given way to fall, and the last piece of my Seattle life had flown away.

Later, I would come to empathize with Nick. My health crisis was a lot to mix into a carefree post-college relationship. And he had struggles of his own. Two pathetic souls do not make great romantic partners. And how attractive can your girlfriend be when she's sporting a wig, machine dependent, and tubed up? (Here's a dating tip: Don't let your tubes hang loose.)

I believe now, absent my health crisis, the glue that had connected us in college would still have lost its adhesion. Our bond was more Elmer's than superglue. But at the time, the complicated ending with Nick dealt a powerful punch aided by the muscular force of illness.

After he left, a disturbing dream woke me in the middle of the night. When Steve and I were youngsters, we played with a drugstore toy—a wooden paddle with a ball attached by an elastic string. The goal was to see how many times you could bounce the rubber ball off the paddle. In my dream, I was a ball attached to the world with an elastic string. Every time I contacted the earth's surface, it flung me back into the surrounding dark space. Unseen forces made it impossible for me to land. I woke, sat upright, and stared blankly into the darkness. I felt complete rejection—not just by my Seattle existence, not just by Nick, not just by my body's betrayal, but by the entire world.

26.

Waiting List

MY LONELINESS SPURRED MEMORY REPLAYS OF MY LIFE in Seattle. I thought about when a robbery spooked Lisa and me to move out of our first apartment with Cindy, and we rented a U-Haul truck. Jamming it with our stuff, we motored off to our new place.

Not long before the move, Lisa tried to teach me how to drive her stick shift in an empty parking lot. The car violently jerked while I tried to connect an action to her words that syncopated with each jolt. "Clutch!" Lurch. "Clutch!" Lurch. "Clutch!" Lurch.

That's why she was the chosen driver of the rented stick shift truck. As we trudged up the steep hill of the Queen Anne neighborhood toward apartment #303, the crudeness of the clunky vehicle became apparent. While Lisa attempted to balance the release of the brake with the gas pedal, we slid backward on the hill.

"You're going backward!" I screamed. Unnecessarily. She already knew that.

"I can't drive this truck!" Lisa barked as she leaned forward with a death grip on the plastic steering wheel. We rolled toward the car behind us. She finally found the clutch's sweet spot and slowly inched the truck up the hill. We burst into hysterical laughter.

"Did you see," I said, doubled over, laughing through my words, "how close we came to hitting that guy?"

"Well, you're of no use. You can't even drive the damn truck," Lisa said through her anxious smile. The adrenaline-fueled moment came and went. We shared a full-on hearty laugh in the aftermath of our relief because disaster averted—we made it up that hill.

I thought about that moment a lot as I chugged through my dialysis sessions. It made me happy to remember how Lisa and I forged slowly upward, transitioning from scared to joyful, and inching toward independence in the world that awaited us. When I ruminated on how I was going to move forward, I remembered that shaky but steady climb of the truck like the little engine that could.

My visualizations continued. Buoyant pink bubbles wrapped me in good health and raised me into a blue sky. Bright lights spilled from my heart like an inner sun that connected to the sun on the horizon. Imagined illumination filled me with hope for a transplant.

Meanwhile, my brother Steve moved back home to start a marketing job for a specialty line of food products. It was a temporary pit stop as he figured out what he wanted to do "with the rest of his life." Despite his uncertainty, I wanted to live vicariously and hear stories about his new job. I envied his excellent health, employment, and ability to be normal in the world. But he didn't see it that way.

"You know," Steve said one night as we sat in the family room, "since I've graduated from college, I feel a lot of pressure about my future and how everything will work out. Isn't it everyone's worst fear that they'll be unmarried at thirty-five?" I could see agitation in his face as he tensed his lips.

"I'll be married at thirty-five," I stated forcefully, leaning forward in my chair.

"What?" Steve looked straight at me and widened his eyes. "How can you be sure of that?" His tone clarified that he thought my statement was a long shot.

I snapped back, "Well, of course I'll be married by then."

"Um . . . not to be rude, but considering what's going on with your health, your confidence is surprising. It wouldn't hurt to add a dose of reality into that mix." His eyebrows raised.

I took issue with his concept of "reality." What's reality, anyway? You can't project a guess onto the future and call it reality. The way I saw it, the future is a movie people direct inside their heads. So I preferred to produce a show with a happy ending. Jeez. Didn't he get it? I was steeped in the laws of attraction!

"I admire your denial," he said, shaking his head.

His half-smile provoked me. "Denial of what? There is no preordained proclamation that I won't get married," I said with elevated volume. My defensive pep talk was underway. *Don't question the way your life will unfold; powerful thoughts are on your side!* But resentment stirred in my gut as my shoulders tightened into knots. This was messed up. Steve's life was good. He had his health. Didn't he realize its value?

I didn't know then what I know now. My health problems didn't disqualify Steve from having issues of his own. There's no contest for life's problems. Everyone has something. But I'll admit, at twenty-three, I felt quicksand pulling me under while everyone else remained on solid ground. Maybe I jumped on Steve's doubts about marriage and the future because buried below my cultivated confidence, I had the same fears.

It was November 1988. The leaves had fallen from the trees and winter circled back around. A year had passed since my diagnosis, and I'd been on dialysis for six months.

"It's time," Dr. Brown said at my appointment. Mom, my reliable sidekick, sat by my side. "Now that you have six months of dialysis under your belt, you're much stronger, and a good candidate for transplantation." I took a deep breath and felt my shoulders drop with relief as I hit this milestone in my waiting game. "It could take up to three years to receive a kidney," he explained, to manage my expectations. "But some patients receive a kidney within one to two years. There is no way of knowing."

I was approaching my twenty-fourth birthday in December, so if his three-year time frame was correct, well, you can do the math. Was I to lose the years from twenty-two to twenty-seven before I could reclaim my life? That was a crushing thought. So I focused on day by day by day by day by day by day by day.

"What about family members?" Dr. Brown asked. "We know living donor transplants are best. Perhaps a member of your family would consider donation."

"I would," Mom said immediately. She straightened up and moved forward.

"Wait! What?" I blurted out. As if injected with a jolt of caffeine, my heart quickened. I whipped my head sideways to look at Mom.

"Let's start with blood type. Liz, do you know yours?" he asked.

"I'm A, Larry is B, and Steve is AB," she said, like she was reciting the ages of family members. She had looked into this, although I didn't know it.

"You're the only compatible one," Dr. Brown continued. "Your blood type A is the same as Jennifer's." I looked back and forth as if they were playing Ping-Pong.

I pushed myself forward to the edge of my seat and raised my hands to conduct their conversation. "Slow down," I said.

"Jennifer, there is a simple antigen blood test that determines if it's even possible." Dr. Brown explained. He suggested we explore it because if my mom and I were a match, we would avoid the wait list.

After our blood tests came back, the transplant center quickly confirmed sweet and bitter results: I was a suitable candidate for transplant, but Mom and I did not have enough matching antigens for compatibility. We had no way of knowing this possibility would circle back in the years to come.

But thank goodness, now I was on the list.

The United Network for Organ Sharing (UNOS) manages this considerable list with a computerized network. This is how it works: When a kidney becomes available, UNOS matches it to those who are waiting. Naturally, it won't be a match for everyone. So they generate a ranked, suitable subset of potential recipients.

Various criteria (medical compatibility, medical urgency, the distance between the kidney and the person who needs it, the organ size, and time on the list) are evaluated to determine the best candidate. The lucky candidate must be "healthy" (so to speak) and ready for immediate surgery. If the first guy or gal has the flu or a cold, for example, they rule him or her out, and the kidney goes to the next suitable recipient. At some undetermined point, that suitable recipient would be me.

All I had to do was wait. Thinking back, my life segmented into various chunks of time endurance. I've learned that time is such a cunning and devious partner; it passes so quickly when you are not paying attention, or when you don't want it to—yet ever so slowly when you do.

At least the dialysis run was quantifiable; I could track it down to the finish. If only I could observe a digital display of my transplant countdown. I wanted to replace the uncertainty with something tangible, something I could see.

The clinic assigned me a transplant coordinator, Mary, and a black beeper with a hook on the back for secure attachment. They instructed me to always carry it (these were pre–cell phone days) so I would be instantly reachable. It was my constant reminder to hurry up and wait. And hope on. So I visualized hearing the beep from that box that would restore my life.

27.

Lucky List

IN DECEMBER, I TRAVELED TO MY FRIEND KRISTIN'S wedding in Boulder. In college, she had been the Pi Phi president while I held the humorously named position of vice president of moral advancement. (No joke. Moral advancement is a tall order.) The job involved things like alcohol awareness seminars, conducting reviews with the executive committee, and overall sorority business.

Kristin had met Pete on campus, and they'd been dating for years, so when she called to say they were getting married, the announcement didn't surprise me. When she asked if I would be a bridesmaid, I felt honored.

Travel was tricky with my schedule. Because of the whirlwind that had transpired since I flew back to Minneapolis just over a year earlier, I hadn't gone many places. But I planned to fly to Boulder on Friday night, after my treatment, and return home Sunday night. If my dear friends were getting married, nothing would stop me from being there.

The transplant clinic reminded me to always keep my beeper with me. If a kidney became available, I would take the first flight back.

My hair had grown back with a mind of its own. It was curly, slightly red, and unwieldy. So I invested in hair extensions to bridge the difference. With my glossy brunette strands, I looked and felt like a sort-of-normal girl.

At first, nerves overcame me, and I worried about seeing everyone. I felt like no one would really understand what I'd been through, like it was a shameful secret. So I spent most of the flight biting my lower lip and battling anxious thoughts. Yet when I first absorbed Kristin's and Pete's ginormous, uncontained smiles, my out-of-place fears fell away.

At the groom's dinner, I met a friend of Pete's who was in medical school. Like an eager student, he seemed fascinated by my recent experiences. As we sat together at a bar, I whipped out the pamphlet from my purse that summarized my fluid recommendations. My favorite part suggested alcohol be consumed as shots, to reduce fluid ounces. We both chuckled. Then he shouted with mock authority to the bartender, "Doctor's orders. Get the lady some shots!"

At the end of the night, he kissed me. He tried to put his hand through my hair, but it got hung up on the extension attachments. When I explained the chunky clumps, he said, "Oh wow, I just thought you used a lot of hair gel." I couldn't stop laughing.

Kristin's wedding made me feel fun and attractive for the first time in what seemed like forever. I flew back to Minneapolis on Sunday, buoyed by the weekend and teased by feelings that I could be a cute girl at a party. Despite my beeper, fake hair, and fluid and diet restrictions, despite being tethered to a life-saving machine and the medical world and parental dependence, I could fold into the mix of the other twentysomethings for an exhilarating weekend. And when the celebrations were complete, I'd be back in my hospital chair on Monday.

Monday came quickly. When I walked into the unit, I passed a snoring Olga and then greeted Brad, who looked deflated and sad. He was two years older than my twenty-four years, another patient whose youth shined like neon in the dark. Handsome, medium-brown hair, glasses, with an average-sized build in good shape. His dad had kidney disease (a different affliction from FSGS), and Brad's doctor had recently diagnosed him with the same condition. A married father to a young son, Brad managed his employment hours by working nights and weekends to accommodate his dialysis.

"Over here," Tom called as he prepped my machine, waving.

I walked over to my chair. "Brad seems a little off today."

"Yes. He's struggling with this process," Tom said.

"He handles so much with all this medical stuff, his family, and his job. It must be tough. I really feel for him."

"And how are you doing?" Tom asked. "You've got a lot going on too."

"I don't have the same amount on my plate. And I feel fortunate to have so much support." (Of course, it didn't hurt that I'd just enjoyed a weekend reconnecting with friends in Colorado and kissed a cute guy.) I'd been focusing on my "lucky list"—my supportive parents, good friends, and an excellent doctor. Plus, I was lucky to have health insurance and a college degree. And a roof over my head. I could see movies. And read. And write. And fit into my clothes and see my ankles and tell jokes and have small doses of coffee (espresso did the trick) and enjoy interesting conversations and connect with people and laugh until my stomach hurt. I told myself the essence of what I needed in life was all around me, despite the machine that kept me alive.

"I see a lot of patients," Tom said, "and some do better than others. Attitude matters. No matter what you deal with, keep that positive outlook. It will help you." It was not revolutionary advice. Nobody walks around saying, "Here's a little-known tip, be super negative." But as it often goes with things we already know, words sound more substantial when delivered via someone else.

I recited this lucky list while I closed my eyes, and the treatment began. This thought train took me to a happy place. And like a sister to creative visualization, focusing on the good-in-the-now helped me.

"You slipped on fluid this time," Tom said as he programmed my machine. "I'll set the goal to remove it all, but if you have any cramping or feel light-headed, let me know right away."

"Those darn commercials," I replied, using Olga's favorite excuse. The extra fluid I'd had over the weekend had added up. And I feared the price I'd now pay for my indulgence in feeling "normal" for a few days.

"I drink lots of coffee," Hazel, who sat to my left, remarked in a high, soft voice. She was watching Tom as he started my run. A decade younger than Olga, Hazel was typically quiet.

"You like coffee?" I asked.

"Oh yes. I can't do anything anymore. I can hardly eat what I want. I don't have sex no more. I can't get myself drunk. So believe me, you know what I do? I drink coffee."

"Yeah, it's good to have something, Hazel," I responded.

Tom looked at me and whispered, "Is coffee a replacement for sex?" He wasn't making fun of her, just joking around. She presented an unusual juxtaposition between the two "vices," but I knew what she meant.

I admired Hazel's effort to find something that made her happy. Instead of using her life lemons to make lemonade, she brewed Folgers. I liked that. Coffee made it onto her lucky list. I had developed a keen appreciation for small wonders that make big bummers better.

About an hour into the run, a pang suddenly screamed from my foot. "Tom!" I tried to raise my voice to reach him from across the room, but it came out high and weak. Thank goodness, he heard me. Cramping was often the result of pulling too much fluid too fast. I might regret my weekend shenanigans after all.

Tom ran over. "I'll lower the fluid rate," he said. The cramp relentlessly clamped onto my foot and ascended to my lower calf. I grimaced as I flexed my foot to stretch the stronghold of the tightened muscle.

"Hold on," Tom instructed, pushing buttons. The cramp reversed and overtook the top of my foot and the front of my calf. So I wiggled my foot, pointing, flexing, but the pain accelerated to excruciating. My head felt light, and my brain fogged over.

"Tom . . . I'm going to pass out," I said as a cold clamminess beaded my face.

"Help here!" Tom shouted. Mark ran over and pushed my chair to a full recline and took my blood pressure. Tom shut off the pumps and opened the saline line for a quick infusion of fluid. I wiggled my toes to keep myself from floating off.

"This saline infusion will help," Tom assured me. "Your blood pressure is crashing."

"Eighty-six over forty-four," Mark said.

The fluid pumped in, and the cramp's dissipation began. "It's getting better," I said, my voice a whisper.

"Ninety-nine over fifty-five," Mark reported after he took another blood pressure reading.

"Glad you're coming back to us," Tom said, still focused on my blood pressure and getting more fluid into my system. "You okay?"

"Yeah, yeah, yeah. It's definitely better, but I feel wiped."

"That'll knock you out for the day. Pulling that much fluid is very difficult on your body. That's why you crashed."

My body stabilized. The cramps let go, and my blood pressure rose. But I still felt like a truck had smashed me. I sat in the chair for a while afterward until I finally felt ready to get up.

As I was leaving, Tom double-checked my steadiness. "I'm fine, Tom," I said, and offered a weak smile. "But it might take me a day or two before I view today's run with a positive attitude."

This notion of positivity, if I had it as Tom suggested, may have stemmed from Dad's start-living techniques and his dedication to Dale Carnegie. In that spirit, Dad created a family tradition when Steve and I were young—the report card reward. After a satisfactory grade review, the four of us went to Bridgeman's Ice Cream Parlor to celebrate.

Mom loved peppermint bonbon. Steve went for the old-fashioned vanilla malt served in a big fluted glass (with that bonus overflow in a metal container), and Dad chose a hot fudge sundae. I picked the sampler—an excessive presentation of many flavors and toppings in an ice cube tray.

Supposedly, good work comprised the criteria for this tradition. But my dad skipped the grade review as the tradition continued. So I asked, "What would you have done if we'd bombed our report cards?"

"I guess then I'd limit you to just one scoop," he replied with a chuckle. Report cards were just the excuse; these ice cream outings were celebrations of "just because." There is loveliness in that. This memory, being a free and easygoing kid spooning up whipped cream, reminded me of easy-access joy.

Like Hazel's coffee and my bonus cranberry juice, unremarkable things could offer quiet joy every day while I waited on the list. I carried that spirit forward as my lucky list helped bridge the gap until my transplant.

28.

Ida

IT BECAME SPRING OF 1989. MY MEDICAL STUDENT kiss briefly tamped down the fear I'd be alone forever, and my affirmations included images of being with someone. But my love life was uneventful—unless I counted Elliott from dialysis.

Mild-mannered and quiet, Elliott had started dialysis treatments in his twenties too. Although I wanted to be his friend, he was interested in more. It felt awkward when he'd show up during my treatment as my blood pressure dropped and I wanted to sleep.

I explained to Lisa during a phone conversation, "I'm worried Elliott figures we'd be a good fit since we're both young with bum kidneys." I cradled the phone between my ear and shoulder, sitting on my bed.

"So he just comes and sits there while you're hooked up?"

"Yes! And I have nowhere to go. I tell him I'm tired and close my eyes. He'd stay the entire time and watch me sleep if I didn't ask him to leave. It's uniquely stressful." I felt my shoulders bunch up as I worried that I'd hurt his feelings.

"Oh, no . . . did he ask you out?"

"Not yet. I know how much it sucks being on dialysis, and he's a nice guy, but I don't want to date him. Am I terrible?" I asked.

"I don't think dialysis in common requires you to date the guy, Jen."

Elliott probably considered us compatible because we were defective merchandise. This was a distressing thought. Nick's comments about me being a "freak" circled back again. Did Elliott think of himself as a freak? Did he think we were both damaged goods? I wondered if being alone was my best option, because that way I wouldn't disrupt another life with my problems. The thought hit me as logical and exceedingly lonely.

Before I was torn from the Velcro that attached me to the Pacific Northwest, lonely thoughts didn't populate my mind. My college campus was extrovert heaven. I remembered my daily walk down the evergreen needle–covered walkways to the library, passing friends and acquaintances. *Hi. See you this weekend? Are you ready for the test?* It was like living in a city of people my age, all hungry for connection. We soaked each other up like sponges. And Nick and Lisa were my constant companions. I'd felt whole then.

At dialysis one afternoon, Sue, the social worker, stood before me with her caring smile. "How are you dealing with this dialysis business?" she asked.

"Okay?" I said hesitantly. "I'm not sure how to answer that question."

"I think you're doing great. But dialysis is tough. I suggest patients ease into the adjustment with help from a psychologist," she explained. "You have a wonderful attitude. Still, you've had a significant event change a lot of things in your life, and it's normal to seek guidance on how to cope with that. I'll give you a referral, and you decide." She handed me a piece of paper.

"Thanks, Sue," I said, taking the sheet. She had circled a name, Ida, and a phone number. I wasn't sure how a psychologist would help me, but I was willing to try it, just as I'd been willing to try an arm puller and the music man.

A week later, I ventured out to learn how to "adjust" to my

damaged life. I drove to Loring Park, that charming area bordering downtown Minneapolis with a mix of apartments, restaurants, walking paths, and Ida's office.

I sank into a spongy brown love seat. *How many people have sat here for adjustment?* Ida was a petite, thick woman with a strong German accent, and had received background on my health from Sue. I set aside my lucky-list thinking and talked about the challenges I faced, starting with the fluid restrictions.

"I'm so thirsty all the time. I have obscene dreams about drinking tons of water," I explained. She listened. She nodded. She looked like Dr. Ruth.

"You should go to AA meetings," Ida said. She wore a smug look of self-satisfaction.

"Why?" I asked, confused. "I don't have a problem with alcohol."

"Ah, but you have a drinking problem of sorts," she said. "You are fluid restricted, and those in AA are alcohol restricted. You share a common bond." She seemed pleased with this clever psychological improvisation. That "bond" she referenced did *not* strike me as a common one, so I involuntarily scoffed out loud. Yet she was quite serious.

I thought it was an odd recommendation. The suggestion to drink alcohol shots (from my trusty fluid management pamphlet) flashed through my mind. I imagined being that rare AA attendee trying to explain that I blew it and chugged two huge glasses of ice water. If only I had knocked back two small shots of vodka instead. Needless to say, I did not seek an AA meeting.

Despite that not-so-great idea, I continued our sessions. Each week, I sank into Ida's couch of misery and revealed my thoughts. She stared at me intensely. I focused on her gray bun and small, stocky frame. She looked tiny in her big swivel chair because her feet didn't quite touch the ground.

"I don't feel like I'm part of the world," I complained. "I want a job. I do nothing."

She responded directly, "Jennifer, dialysis is not 'nothing.' This procedure is keeping you alive and takes a lot of time and energy. You're brave. Don't belittle yourself. You do more than most just to stay healthy."

"Dialysis is something. A whole lot of something. But it's so far from the right thing. I just don't feel like it's enough," I said, exasperated. "There must be more to this story. There must be more to me."

"Give yourself a break," she replied. "Be patient. You gain nothing from telling yourself that you 'do nothing.' It's simply inaccurate," she stated forcefully.

My thoughts spun wildly from resisting the identity of freakishness to appreciating my lucky list, to longing for unlimited ice water, to pining for a job. As I dreamed of living like all my friends, I seized with fear—what if I wouldn't be able to achieve a meaningful life?

29.

Die Young

SOON AFTER, THE DIALYSIS MACHINE HUMMED AS IT removed toxins from my blood. Semi-reclined in my chair, covered with a blanket, drowsiness began to overtake me. As my eyes flittered between open and shut, I saw Elliott approach. "Oh, hey. How are you doing?" I asked.

"Fine . . . you know." He shrugged his shoulders and half smiled. He rolled a stool over and sat by my side. Continuing to chat and compare health notes, he said, "I'm twenty-three. How old are you?"

"I'm twenty-four," I responded. My effort to smile felt weak.

"An older woman, I like that." He rubbed his fingertips together and looked down in a shy retreat. Except for the brown color of his curly locks, he looked like he'd be well cast as Napoleon Dynamite's brother. "Sorry, that was weird." His cheeks flushed with pink.

"That's okay," I said, trying to ease his discomfort.

"There aren't a lot of young people around here," he continued, spinning in his stool to look around the room.

"Yeah, we are definitely the young ones." Pressing my lips together, I widened my eyes in agreement.

"You're really pretty. I like the scarves you wear." His soft tone picked up volume, but again, he looked down.

The awkwardness kicked up a notch, and a cloak of discomfort wrapped around me. "Thanks. You're friendly to visit, but

I'm so tired. Do you ever feel exhausted during your run—like you need to close your eyes?"

"Sure. Don't worry. I'll just sit here."

As he stared at me, the idea of him sitting silently while I dozed off made me uneasy. "Elliott, I don't want to be rude, but I might fall asleep," I said.

"Oh, okay. I understand. I'll stop by again for another visit." Relieved, I lowered my lids, and Elliott left.

Well into my next treatment, I glanced over to the waiting area and saw Elliott walking in. He waved and came right over. Cutting right to the chase, he said, "Do you want to go out with me sometime?" His hands in his pockets, he rocked side by side on his feet. As I considered what to say, he populated the space with more words. "I'll show you my new car. It's nice."

Oh, no. Silent stall. I focused on the car and asked, "Did you just buy it?" Truth is, I was put off by his approach. Technicians had strapped me to a blood-sucking machine—talk about a captive audience! It just wasn't the ideal time to field date requests.

"Yeah, it's new." He didn't glance down this time; today he seemed unwavering and looked straight at me.

"Tell me about it," I said. Second stall.

"It's midnight blue, and the control panel's cool." He lit up talking about his new wheels. And it was endearing, as if he was a boy bragging about a new bike. He usually broadcast a downtrodden gaze, so I enjoyed seeing his eyes brighten. I had to answer his question now (a three-question stall would be flat-out rude), but I was afraid to hurt his feelings.

"A lot is going on for me right now, Elliott. I broke up with my boyfriend not too long ago, and I don't really want to go out on dates."

"Oh," he said, averting my eyes and pausing for a few seconds. "Well, I just thought it would be nice to have a girlfriend that understands all this stuff." He gestured around the room full of patients, technicians, machines, and nurses. "I think it's hard, don't you?" he asked.

"Yeah, it sucks. This isn't what I figured I'd be doing, that's for sure."

Then he said, "It's such a bummer we're going to die young."

Excuse me? His words caught me off guard. I had seen the date request coming, but not the death pronouncement. I wanted to run away, but again, since I was tethered to a machine, that impulse was impossible. My cheeks burned.

"Don't you wonder what will happen . . . when we die?" he continued.

As my blood pumped through the machine, my heart pumped faster too. *I'm not going to die on dialysis, Elliott. Dr. Brown never presented death as a possibility.* I wasn't immune to his thoughts, but he made it sound as if death lurked around the corner.

"No. I don't like to think about that," I responded. "I like to focus on how grateful I am for the things I have; it makes me feel better. You know? There are two ways to look at it. From one perspective, dialysis is horrible. But the other view is that dialysis keeps us alive. I'm grateful for that."

"Yeah, I guess," he replied, as he considered my dialysis-is-life conversation twister. "Still, it's hard not to think about it," he said. His face fell, and I wanted to melt for him. Pain spilled from his pores while his shoulders slumped.

"We're alive today, Elliott, right here and now. Consider how you can make this situation better and visualize a happy path forward." I knew I sounded like an insufferable self-help book, but I believed in what I said. I had assimilated some of

Dad's stop-worrying techniques and channeled thoughts about death toward my determination to live.

"Sure, I guess. I'll let you sleep." Elliott left.

I shut my eyes and felt guilty for rebuffing his advances. As I worried about him, I worried about myself too. I didn't want to go down a negative path. My work-in-progress positivity was fragile, and despite my efforts to ignore them, Elliott's words played as unwelcome background music in my head.

Die young. Die young. Die young. Die young. Die young.

30

Denial Support

IT WAS NOW APRIL 1989, AND I'D BEEN ON DIALYSIS FOR ten months. I sat on my parents' porch one early evening, and a light breeze filtered through the screens. My mom's flowers bloomed brightly in the pots scattered on the adjacent deck.

"What are you reading?" Dad asked as he walked in and joined me.

"Affirmations," I said, while rubbing a cramp out of my lower calf. My cherished glass of ice was on the table next to me.

"How're you feeling?"

"I'm into your theory about accepting the worst, Dad. I don't like it—okay, I hate it— but here I am. So now that I've hit rock bottom, I'm pouring my thoughts into my transplant. That's my future." I had been on visualization overdrive to imagine getting a new kidney.

"Good deal," he said, and sat down in the corner chair to read the paper. Mickey ambled over, spun in a circle until she found the right position, and curled up at his feet.

"The hard part is, I'm stuck. And I'm so bored. I spend all my time at the hospital." Dad set down his *Wall Street Journal*. "I don't have a job. I'm just spinning my wheels."

"I'm sorry about all this," he said. I knew he'd take it all away if he could.

"Come to think of it, this rock bottom is awful. Well, now, just like that . . . I'm in a bad mood." How quickly I transitioned from hopeful to pissed off. If I'd been a mood ring, my color would've transitioned into black.

"I realize it's hard, Jenny. Give it time. You'll get a good job when this evens out."

Mom walked in and joined the conversation. "What about a support group?" she asked. "I saw a sign at the dialysis unit about a group for patients and family. It might help if you talked to some other people in your situation."

"I guess." I wasn't enthusiastic.

"Let's give it a try. I'll go with you?" she suggested. "Come on . . ." She raised her eyebrows and paused—and I knew exactly what she was about to say.

"You and your riots," I laughed. "Okay, let's try it."

The following Tuesday night, Mom and I found the sign by a room near the unit: PATIENT AND FAMILY DIALYSIS SUPPORT GROUP. About ten seated people between the ages of forty to sixty-five gathered in a circle. Understandably, they did not look like a joyful bunch.

I don't want to be here. I realized that thought ran through my mind just about everywhere lately. We went around the circle and introduced ourselves by name, diagnosis, dialysis start date, and who was with us. "Hi, I'm Jennifer. I have focal sclerosis, and I have been on dialysis since June. This is my mom."

I hated saying that; I hated identifying myself with this illness and this treatment. I wanted so much more than this. And yet here I was, meeting people who projected the future I wanted to reject.

A mother and her daughter sat across from Mom and me. This woman was in her early forties. Her teenage daughter slumped low in her seat as if an invisible weight pressed her down. The woman spoke in a monotone voice and said she'd been dialyzing for a year and a half. She pushed a piece of her dull, gray-streaked hair from her gaunt face. Her skin had an unnatural yellow-brown tone.

Her haunted expression scared me. Her energy, hollow and depressed, seemed inaccessible, as if she'd dropped into a void. I didn't want to fall into that void. Was this what was ahead for me?

She and the other attendees held cups of coffee and shared dialysis difficulties. I had so much in common with them: the blood pressure drops, fluid and food restrictions, cramps, and nausea, yet I stared at the floor. These people seemed well versed in despair. As I did when I saw the words *morbidity* and *mortality* in the biomedical library and when I repelled Elliott's death talk, I wouldn't allow myself to take this on.

I couldn't commiserate or give in to discouragement because that's not how I wanted to see myself. Support groups are helpful when you accept you need support. Perhaps I wanted denial support more than dialysis support. Is that a thing? A group where everyone says it's not that bad? Looking back, I realize my denial wasn't unproductive; it was a determined focus to view my situation as a pit stop on the way to a transplant—and the resurrection of my rightful healthy life.

Although I knew I didn't choose this reality, I could choose the way I thought about it. Between hope and despair, hope was more comfortable to wear. Despair was ill-fitting. Being here reinforced that I wasn't normal. I wanted to preserve my positivity and optimistic armor. I feared this support group would pierce my protection.

But what about Mom? I wince now to think maybe *she* needed the support group. What private conversations did she share with my dad? Did they hide their anguish from me? (Years later, Mom told me she found a moment alone during the worst of it. Unleashing a deep aching sound, she couldn't believe the noise was her own. The wail carried through the empty house. When I asked her what it sounded like, she replied, "A primal scream.")

When the meeting finished, everyone dispersed. Mom turned and said, "What did you think?"

"That was depressing as hell. That lady with her daughter seemed really sick and miserable. What did you think, Mom?"

"There was a lot of sadness there," she agreed.

"Do I seem like those people?" I asked.

"Well, do you feel miserable?"

"Yeah, I guess. I'm pretty miserable too, but no . . . not like that. I don't want to be like that." Pushing it away, I didn't have the depth yet to understand life holds joy and despair, and it's okay to feel a variety of emotions. Instead, I said, "This is not forever for me. This is a temporary state. I just need to hang on until I get my transplant."

31.

Seattle, Again

I DIDN'T WANT TO EMBRACE DESPAIR. INSTEAD, I visualized returning to my youthful life in Seattle—my healthy, happy self, boarding a flight bound for Sea-Tac Airport . . . stepping off the plane, welcomed by friends, restored and ready to pick up where I'd left off. The image was vivid. I smelled the evergreen aroma of pine. I saw the sparkling waters of Puget Sound. I tasted the robust, dark-roasted coffee. I enjoyed the wind and humid air on my face. And I heard the unified gales of laughter from Lisa, Cindy, Susan, and Gillian.

This mental movie (inspired by *Creative Visualization*) eased my profound sense of alienation. The image constructed a bridge from despair to hope. I'd been in Minneapolis for almost a year and a half, on dialysis for a year, and accrued six months on the transplant list. Would I ever get back to Seattle?

One night, Mom, Dad, and I sat down on the family room sofa. "I keep thinking," I started and paused, knowing my parents would not like my forthcoming idea. My mom looked at me curiously. "I keep thinking I will move back to Seattle when this is all done, but the wait is so long. I think I should move back to Seattle now while I wait for a transplant."

Both of their eyes grew wide. "Jenny, that's crazy," Mom said. "You will dialyze there?"

"I want to," I responded.

"Where?"

"There's a social worker who can place me in a unit close to the house."

"What house?" they both asked simultaneously.

"Cindy and Susan rent a house in the University District. There's an extra room I can use. The rent divided by three is cheap. Maybe I can find writing jobs and go back to school for a while."

The plan sounded brilliant to me. Yes, I'd have treatments three times a week, but I'd be back in the city I'd considered my home. And I'd be back with my friends.

"I think it's a bad idea. What if you have complications and need to be hospitalized? There's no Dr. Brown there. You'll need a new nephrologist," Mom said in a higher than usual voice. "And there's no family there. This doesn't seem to be the right time. What if a kidney becomes available?"

"The transplant center will call or buzz me with this beeper," I replied, patting my constant companion hooked on my belt loop. "I'm trying to speed up the waiting process."

"Why is this so important to you?" Dad asked.

"Because I need to have my life back." The words flew out fast and high-pitched. I paused to collect myself. "I feel stuck here, and it seems like I'll never get a kidney. Something good needs to happen. I want to feel like me again. Just for the summer." I was vying for understanding. "Please, I need to do this."

Being fully supported by my parents at my age was like having training wheels back on my bike. I needed to reconnect with my friends and handle my medical mess without my parents' steady presence. If I couldn't be independent with full-time employment just yet, at least I needed to navigate my illness independently, in some form.

"I'm so sorry for all of this," I said, hating that I heaped onto their mountain of concern.

Dad let out a breath. "Well, try it and see."

"Clearly, I can't talk you out of it," Mom said, getting up and leaving the family room. I followed her into the kitchen and gave her a hug.

"Do you understand?" I asked. She was my riot buddy; I appreciated her so much and didn't want to cause her more distress. But at the same time, I felt Seattle would restore me.

"I understand," she said. "Worry is worry. I can worry long distance, I suppose."

"It'll be okay," I said with determination and firm conviction. I was about to take a step toward reclaiming my life.

By the summer of 1989, I was back in Seattle. Susan and Cindy were my new roommates, and Lisa lived close by. We picked up seamlessly from where we'd left off. I felt age appropriate again, a twentysomething with friends, unattached, ready to be back in the world, free-spirited and easygoing, despite keeping a careful eye on my fluids and foods and showing up for dialysis.

We shared party talk, current or past boyfriend details, career frustrations, progress, updates on our college cohorts, gossip on who was doing what to whom, and who worked where and why. Nick had moved to California, so I didn't have to face that situation, thank goodness.

When I was away, Lisa's sister had used my car. So my transportation was already set. My first step was to meet the social worker at the Swedish Medical Center in the Capitol Hill area. This was close to the apartment Lisa, Cindy, and I had lived in before that robbery ruined the experience. The thief broke in, stole loads of stuff, and scattered condoms all around. We came home to discover this condom-confetti mess. Our burglar was either super creepy or adamant about encouraging safe sex. Probably super creepy.

A guy named Matt greeted me at the medical center. He led me to his small office to discuss my placement options for dialysis treatment facilities. He was in his thirties and had a laid-back vibe—corduroy pants, slightly crumpled white oxford shirt, and brown hair that looked overdue for a cut that was unlikely a priority. "There is a unit relatively close," he said hesitantly. He sat behind a desk, and a window to his right looked over a busy street named Broadway. "I should warn you, it's a different crowd that dialyzes there, and it's hard for me to imagine that you'd fit in," he continued. His eyes won me over; he looked like he cared.

"Why?" I asked. Did he not realize I had befriended Olga and Hazel and shared space with various dialysis patients? "It was a bit shocking when I first started," I said, "but I know what it's like now."

"This is not the same," he explained. "When I say a different crowd, I mean a tough crowd—prison inmates. Many of them are shackled to their chairs."

"Well, okay then," I said. "Let's skip that one." *Come on now, Matt, was that even worth bringing up?* I wasn't interested in layering a "tough crowd" over the general bummer of treatment.

"Have you thought about peritoneal dialysis?" he asked. "This option eliminates the three-times-a-week clinic visit. Instead, you dialyze yourself by filling your abdominal cavity with cleansing fluid through a tube. The peritoneum acts as the membrane that exchanges the fluids and toxins. Waste products are absorbed into the fluid and then discarded."

"Wow, no clinic?" That sounded like a plus.

"No clinic. The drawback of this procedure is that your abdomen could become distended," Matt explained. "Young women sometimes avoid this treatment because the large fluid exchanges can make it look like you're pregnant."

Matt was now two for two. So far, his ideas sucked. My developed fistula looked like a large winding snake tucked under the surface of my skin on my left arm. I'd been disfigured enough, thank you. "Those are not great choices," I said. "What else can you do for me? Because hanging out with prison inmates or looking pregnant are not appealing options."

"Let's see what clinics may have room for you near the University of Washington."

Matt made calls, pulled strings, and found an acceptable alternative dialysis center in the University District near our home. I began treatments there.

The first time, I met Laurie, a golden-blonde nurse in spruce-green scrubs. She greeted me with warmth and admired my fistula. "I'll have no problem sticking your access; it's beautiful."

"I'm glad you think so," I said. *Not the word I'd use to describe it.*

The machine was the same, but the atmosphere was different. No patients sat close by, no Olgas shouted bizarre commentary, no Hazels complained, no Brads commiserated. The doctors extended my treatment to three and a half hours because longer runs were easier on the body.

I enrolled in communications and psychology classes at the University of Washington to stimulate my brainpower. I was older than the other students in the summer class by about three years, but the difference I felt between our perspectives wasn't because of age. My private life-and-death activity on the side colored my view. I had a shameful medical secret tucked away, and it poked at me like a stick of self-consciousness. I felt different from these students because I imagined they had their invincibility shields intact. I didn't know them, but I wanted to be them. They seemed so perfect and problem free. I had not yet fully learned that no one's life is problem free, and perfection is impossible.

I continued to wake up nauseous in the mornings, but a bit of toast made it better. I committed to ice cubes and the recommended diet, and I loved being with Cindy, Susan, Gillian, and Lisa. My comfort friends. Being a part of their lives again brought me the connection that I'd longed for over the last year and a half.

"Hey," Cindy said one night. "Mark called, and Jack is getting everyone together this weekend." We were lounging in pajamas in the dim family room of our rental home. We sat on used furniture next to beat-up side tables. The carpet was ghastly, and natural light was lacking. Considering it all, it was just right. "Drinks and dancing at a bar," Cindy finished.

"Let's go," Susan replied. Her blue eyes popped against her porcelain skin and brunette bob. Mark and Jack were friends from college.

"I'm in," I said.

The night of the party, I put on a long-sleeved T-shirt, a short cotton skirt, and a pair of sandals.

"I'm going with one of these two shirts," Cindy said as she walked into the living room in her bra. She held up a green patterned sleeveless and a black sleeveless option.

"Black," Susan said. I agreed.

Cindy whipped her blond curly hair into a ponytail. I admired her athletic body; the strength of her legs resembled an anatomy diagram of musculature. Years of playing college basketball were on display, and although I'd never thought about it that much before, I felt jealous of how healthy she was.

But here we were, like we'd been in our sorority housing—comparing outfits, getting dressed, prepping for a social evening. This togetherness felt vital and deeply satisfying. I had started to savor joy. Precious ordinary moments now seemed extraordinary.

I grabbed a rosy lip gloss, rolled on a burst of color, and positioned my sleeve over the bulging fistula. "Let's go."

It was my first party since I'd moved back to Seattle. Once I got past the initial social barrage of caring and kind, "Hey, how are you? Good to see you! I was worried about you! Are you okay?"—I felt like I could be a part of the group once again. Several beers and beverages into the night (lots of ounces for others, a wee bit for me), the dancing began. And the beat of the loud music pulled me onto the dance floor.

I was folding into the mix of the other twentysomethings, feeling buoyed by the music, and enjoying a mini-buzz. Just as I'd experienced at Kristin's wedding, I could still be a young woman at a party. How fun! My anemia still limited my endurance, however, so when I felt short of breath, I sat down to take a break.

"Hey, Jennifer," Jack, the party instigator, said as his tall frame lumbered over and sat down next to me. A foamy beer spilled over the edge of his Solo cup. His blond hair and sporty build broadcast health.

"Hi, Jack, fun party."

"Yeah, it's great to see you. And everyone. So, you're on dialysis, right?" he asked. I told him I'd been having treatments for about a year. "I have a high school friend. His name is Tommy. He's got kidney disease. He was on dialysis too."

I didn't know if the "was" signaled disaster or transplant. With trepidation, I asked, "Really? How's he doing?"

"He's okay. He had a transplant." Jack's eyes kept darting from my face to the dance floor.

"Wow, that's so cool," I said. It was a vicarious thrill to hear of someone off dialysis, living a new life with a fresh kidney. "Waiting is hard. Do you know how long he waited on the list and where he got his kidney?"

"He waited a long time, but I don't know all the details," Jack said, still turning his head back and forth to keep tabs on his guests.

"Hey, Jack!" a jovial guy (beer in his hand, perma-grin) called from across the room. Jack stood to greet his friend and turned to wrap up our conversation. "All I know . . . Tommy's a great guy, and it sucks because he will die so young." Then he walked away.

Not again with this die-young business! His words slapped me. I learned later that Tommy had suffered from illness for most of his life. Maybe this factored into Jack's comment? Even so, his statement felt sharp and confusing. Tommy had reached the holy grail of dialysis alumni, the transplanted person no longer tethered to life by a machine. He'd found the promised land—a new kidney. So why did Jack say that?

I pushed the confusion aside. *I am* not *Tommy. I don't even know Tommy, and I'm going back on that dance floor.*

32

Home?

WE DECONSTRUCTED THE PARTY THE NEXT DAY. "I SAW you talking to Jack," Cindy said.

"Yes, in fact, I had a lovely conversation with Jack about his friend who had a transplant. It concluded with his sorrow about said friend's eventual, hypothetical untimely death."

"What?" Cindy asked.

"You know, we each have our talents, but I have a unique and underappreciated quality—I'm a magnet for death conversations," I replied. "When people see me coming, they pull out their best death material."

"Oh my God, that's not funny," Susan said, giggling. Then we all burst into laughter because first of all, weird, and second, what was the alternative? In our youthful state, death seemed like a naughty word. Laughter came easily, but death was far from our thoughts. The notion of it being tossed out at a party seemed irregular.

Living with Cindy and Susan felt like old times, but I had to reconcile that the times were different. It became increasingly apparent in the vast space between the parties (when everyday life happened). Cindy and Susan had jobs while I sat at dialysis.

One Monday afternoon, a nurse called to warn me about elevated lab results. "Jennifer, your potassium came back high today," the nurse said. "You need to be careful with potassium foods before we see you on Wednesday."

Inner laces tightened inside me. Had I slipped up with high-potassium foods since my last run? I couldn't attribute anything I ate to this elevated level, and high potassium was dangerous. I hadn't explained these details to my friends. So I called home.

Steve answered and bellowed for Mom to pick up the line. As soon as she said hello, I burst into sobs.

"What's going on?" she asked. The concern in her voice felt comforting.

"My potassium is high, and I don't know what I ate. I thought I had done okay. But now I have to watch it." A wild panic came over me. My accumulated anxieties stirred into one big stew.

"How high?" she asked.

"5.9." I squeezed my eyes shut and wrapped the phone cord around my finger.

"Okay, high . . . but you'll be careful. Don't worry too much about it," she replied. Potassium over 6 would trigger a serious alarm, and 5.9 bordered on the edge. But how comforting that she understood this lab value. I didn't need to explain a thing.

Steve had remained on the line. "Wow, Jenny. You're a convincing actress. You seemed fine until Mom got on." Maybe I had become an actress. How many times had I held it together when I wanted to fall apart? I had refined my newfound craft, best actress in a real-life drama.

I remembered a previous high potassium scare in the hospital when Mom climbed into the bed and slept overnight. My fears didn't need to be shaped or filtered with Mom. She saw the raw, real me, stripped of varnish and shine. And she was there even when I was across the country.

That afternoon, I completed class readings and watched an episode of *The Golden Girls*. A Kodak ad played during a commercial break. A young, beautiful bride, fresh-faced and healthy, danced with her tuxedo-clad dad. He beamed. She glowed. The dad flashed back through a series of warmhearted, nostalgic memories—his daughter as an adorable baby, in a kindergarten class, at an elementary school, playing softball, navigating her teenage years. A sweet song played over the series of images with the lyrics of "Daddy's Little Girl."

I'll admit, this was a Hallmark-y commercial if there ever was one, and it threw my amped-up, glossy goals in my face. I wanted my life to resemble this thirty-second snapshot created by Kodak. But it was nothing like this. So I became unhinged. *Damn you, Kodak!*

My mind flooded with memories of the little girl I used to be. The girl who ran to the back door when Dad came home from work and perched on the tops of his feet while he walked into the kitchen. Memories of my mom's crust-free toast and tater tot casserole, my Peggy doll (before Steve drowned her), my Nancy Drew books that came in the mail (via my Nancy Drew book club membership, of course).

I longed to return to the safe bubble of childhood that my parents had created for me. What happened to that once-care-free girl in pigtails?

She was gone.

So was the girl who'd lived in the bubble of invincibility as a twenty-two-year-old in Seattle. What happened to that young woman with a life ahead of her? Had I lost all forms of myself, my past, and my future?

I should have let Cindy and Susan know how alone I felt with my illness. At dialysis. In the house, the city, the state, the world—but I didn't want to be a drag. It was the same lesson I tried to learn from Rachael. I should've embraced that sharing the hard parts doesn't dampen a friendship; it *is* friendship. But I was still trying to rise above it and be closer to some misguided patient-version of perfect.

It was hard work treading water to stay on the surface, and it exhausted me. One evening toward the end of summer, I sat with Cindy and Susan. "My classes are wrapping up soon," I started, "and I think I'll go back to Minneapolis this fall. It seems to be the right place for me to wait out the final stretch. You know how much I've loved reconnecting with you guys this summer."

But like the previous summer with Nick, reality thwarted my intentions to regain normalcy. I pressed up against a hard truth—I was trying to reclaim something that couldn't be reclaimed. I didn't know where I belonged.

My awakened spirituality remained a part of my meditations. I didn't want to lose my connection to the universe and my soul's energy. All the same, my body, here and now, longed for a place to land.

"It'll happen. Hang in there. I'll be sending powerful prayers," Susan said.

"Love you, Jen. I'm praying for that transplant too," Cindy agreed, and initiated an all-in hug.

I dialed the number I knew so well, and my mom answered. "Seattle's run its course, Mom. I'm coming home."

And was I? Going home? I'd spent so much time thinking Seattle was my home and where I should be. But that Seattle didn't exist anymore. I was stuck in place on a treadmill, while my friends ran freely in various directions. I couldn't catch up with them, and they couldn't wait for me. The question became, where was *my* place? Did I really have a home?

33

Still Waiting

SEATTLE DIDN'T RESTORE ME. BACK TO MINNESOTA.
Still waiting. I needed to think forward. My upcoming operation
was the target, and I set my mind on that goal—the promise of
my future attached singularly to a transplant.

I returned to the Abbott dialysis unit with the same cast of
characters. Everyone greeted me with a warm welcome and
asked all about my months in Seattle.

"Be honest," Jerry said. "Our unit is better, right?"

"You know, Jerry, I kind of missed your brand of dialysis.
You guys are all stars." How odd to realize this was the right
place, and how capricious the right place can be. Again and
again, I was learning. A change in perspective makes everything
look different.

During my treatment, I lifted my eyes from my book to see
Sue approaching. She asked me about Seattle, and we chatted.
Then she told me she'd created a newsletter for patients. "Would
you be interested in writing a piece about your experience?"

"Sure," I said. I didn't have to think twice. A task that involved my brain, skills, and a deadline? Basking in the satisfaction of having an assignment, I felt lifted. *Good things will come.*

Weeks later, after the article was published, I shuffled downstairs to relish my three-ounces-of-coffee energy. Mom buttered
her toast and complimented me on the piece. It felt rewarding to
have focused on something professional rather than medical.

Dad chimed in with his stamp of approval. "Well written,

Jenny." He'd spread the paper out in front of him and had already suited up for his workday ahead. "I've been thinking that our office could put your communication and public relations skills to use. Lori is busy with sales, so she can't cover all the communications."

"Are you offering me a job, Dad?" I asked reluctantly, fighting a smile. Was he? I knew he sympathized with my situation, so his proposal might be a blatant act of nepotism/compassion, but it thrilled me.

Dad grinned. He created a position in which I could exercise my skills on Tuesdays and Thursdays (the days free from treatment). And so it began. I worked with his small staff, sent out press releases, answered phones, called subcontractors to pick up plans, wrote drafts of letters to clients, whatever needed doing. From there, I collected rents from tenants (my dad owned the building), developed tenant budgets, and tracked prospective client communications. Not only did that work give me a purpose, but it also eased some feelings of worthlessness and thumb twiddling. And I was once again receiving a paycheck.

Monday, Wednesday, and Friday—go to the clinic for necessary medical procedures. Purpose: to stay alive. Tuesday, Thursday—go to the office to feel like a regular working gal. Purpose: to feel alive.

My high school friends were still in Minneapolis, so I had a social tribe to fall back into when I returned from the Pacific Northwest. There were still parties to attend, things to do, people to hang out with.

Then Rae called one evening after I got home. "I want you to move in with Mike and me," she said. "We rented an apartment on Twenty-Eighth Street, close to the hospital, and it has an extra bedroom. When you're tired after your treatments, you'll practically be home."

Rae had met Mike, her constant companion and soulmate, at the University of Minnesota. His dark hair, tall athletic build, and sharp wit were the ying to the yang of Rae's blond hair, short athletic build, and silly nature.

"I love that idea." Something lifted inside me, knowing that although I missed my Seattle friends, I had friends to live with in Minneapolis too.

"Just know we won't be here that long. It's a temporary pit stop for us," Rachael explained.

"Got it. Is it nice?"

"Well, it is if you like the color brown—it's Brownsville. And the neighborhood is sketchy," she said. "Come see."

Rachael hailed from a half Jewish/half Catholic family. Growing up, my friends and I envied her good fortune to celebrate a variety of holidays, especially Hanukkah and Christmas. Maybe that's why Rachael always carried a spirit of celebration with her; combined with her encouraging nature and refined cooking skills, her personality felt like nourishment.

I drove over to the brown paneled building. Rachael's and Mike's names appeared next to a buzzer on a control panel inside the exterior door. I pushed the button, and Rae jogged down to let me in. "See that corner?" She pointed at the foyer ceiling. "There used to be a security camera there so we could monitor who entered the building."

"Where is it?" I asked.

"Someone stole it," she said as she keyed the door.

"What an ironic theft." Rachael unleashed her lovable cackle.

We walked up a few flights, and she ushered me inside the apartment. "I get what you mean, Rae. Someone has really elevated brown to new heights here." Brown carpet, institution beige-brown walls, and brown laminate, fake-wood kitchen countertops.

"Well?" she asked after she showed me a small square room off the hall beyond the living room.

"It's ideal," I beamed. We tallied my rent portion, wiped dust balls from the baseboards, and I moved in. My parents were happy I was tackling my independence in Minneapolis as opposed to Seattle. And I was too.

"Okay! You're home!" Rae grinned and gripped me in a tight hug.

34

Good Things?

"Hello, honeys," I said one evening as I flung open the apartment door after my treatment. I found Rae and Mike cozied up on the sofa, watching television.

"There she is—all fresh and clean," Mike said. He draped his arm around Rae's shoulder, and she snuggled into his side.

"Hey, Jen, how'd it go?" Rae asked as she straightened up.

"Six pounds flushed down the drain," I replied. Each dialysis session removed the fluid that had built up from the previous session, transforming me from bloated to better.

"I want to get water sucked off me too," Rae said, smiling. "We had a big salty dinner, so we're fat and happy. Can I get you something?"

"No, thanks. I'll pop in a frozen dinner." I grabbed the lean entrée from the freezer and slashed an inch into the plastic covering.

As I loaded it into the microwave, Rae shook her head disapprovingly. "Yuck, what's your flavor tonight?"

"A classic dish of herb roasted chicken," I replied with raised eyebrows, as if it were a delicacy. She rolled her eyes, and I smiled. "I know the protein grams and sodium count, so I'll stick with it."

"At least let me make you some greens?" She didn't wait for an answer. She breezily whipped up a gourmet salad within the five minutes it took to heat the frozen tray of rubbery chicken, white rice, and mushy vegetables.

"How about an ice-cold Diet Coke, Jenny?" Mike presented it as fine champagne. He knew I had a good twelve-ounce fluid allowance after dialysis sucked me dry, so he kept a constant supply of well-chilled beverages in the fridge. "Any dialysis suitors today?" he asked with a wink, handing me the cold can.

"No suitors." I dove into my dinner.

"What was that guy's name again?" he asked.

"Elliott." He'd moved, and I hadn't seen him in months. Despite his unwelcome advances, I cared about him and hoped he was okay.

"Oh, yeah," Mike teased, "the guy who tried to win you over with his new car?" He smiled and elbowed me.

"Don't be mean," I said, although I knew full well that wasn't his motive.

"You know, my grandfather had a car too. He was pretty sexy," Mike added, suppressing a grin. Rachael bumped into his side to stop him from crossing the line with offbeat humor. "It's an odd pickup line, I'm just saying." Mike's eyes twinkled playfully.

Rachael giggled, and I fought back a smile, unsuccessfully, and we all laughed together.

"Seriously, Jen, when you find the right guy, we'll go out on double dates with you." Rae rested her hand on my arm.

"What if Elliott was my only chance?" I asked, suddenly aware that my criteria for a boyfriend, someone I wanted to spend time with, might be too much to ask for under the circumstances. (The medical student at Kristin's wedding was a distant memory.) "I mean, really, maybe it's all I can expect, being sweet-talked about dialysis and death while riding around in a car on a date."

"Oh, please," Rae said.

"You guys, what if my entire life passes me by and there is never another interested Elliott?" I felt pathetic.

"Okay, jokes aside, Jenny, no," Rae said. "You need to find a guy who's an upper, not a downer." Her words brought Michael Jackson to mind. An upper, not a downer. A lover, not a fighter.

"Yeah, I agree," Mike chimed in.

Rae leaned over to kiss Mike on the cheek; perhaps she realized how grateful she was to have found him. I loved their company, friendship, and relationship. It was clear they were headed toward engagement and marriage. They were wonderfully compatible, and I envied their path.

I wanted to be on that path too, but I felt so far from it.

On Tuesdays and Thursdays, my work continued. One day, my dad motioned me into the conference room to meet a well-dressed woman with a commanding presence. "Jennifer, I want to introduce you to Janet Foster. She owns an advertising agency and publishes *New Homes* magazine." I'd seen her before because her office suite was right across the hall.

"Hello, Jennifer. Your dad tells me you worked in public relations in Seattle."

"Yes, at a subsidiary of Ogilvy and Mather," I responded.

"Great national firm. And I hear you've done some writing," Janet continued.

"A little, yes," I replied.

"Janet and her team schedule and design our magazine ads," Dad said. "Lori has been handling this, but she's swamped. It would be helpful if you could take it on. You'll work with Janet and her associate, Wendy. Okay?"

I sat up straight in my chair and felt a burst of energy pulse through me. "Fantastic. I'm thrilled."

"I may have freelance writing opportunities for you too," Janet said. Her hair shined a silver blond, her voice was firm, and she had an imposing stature, easily standing five inches taller than me. The opportunity to work with Janet and Wendy pumped me up. As I immersed myself in their business, I learned so much about advertising, graphic design, copywriting, magazine demographics, and editorial calendars. I recognized that Dad had provided this opportunity, but it was still an opportunity. I gratefully dipped my toe into the business world.

My compartmentalizing nature wanted a tidy separation between being a medical girl on Monday, Wednesdays, and Fridays, and a working girl on Tuesdays and Thursdays. Yet everyone on my dad's staff understood my health situation. That felt okay by me. We were a small-company family. Janet and Wendy also knew I was awaiting a transplant, but we didn't talk about it. I didn't know what to say. I don't think they did either. We seemed confined by the don't-talk-about-illness convention that often thickens the air between acquaintances. They respected my privacy. I guarded my feelings of shame.

We managed a marketing project together and assembled a team to create a corporate brochure. Models posed as a satisfied-client couple, an arrogant photographer captured their image, an artist painted watercolors with a dream-home flavor, and printers made it materialize.

And during the project, I felt painfully self-conscious around the outside professionals. *How do these people see me? Do I look sick? Do they know I'm not normal?* Even so, I tucked those feelings away, plowed forward, and did my job.

The piece received a Marketing and Merchandising Award of Excellence, and I felt jazzed to be part of the team. After that, Janet hired me to write feature articles for her magazine. Definite progress. My love life may have lacked promise, but at work (although it wasn't PR in Seattle) I moved forward on a professional path. My visualizations continued, and I had to continue to believe that good things would come.

35

Movie People

RAE AND MIKE WANTED TO SETTLE INTO A MORE
permanent place about the same time my childhood friend Beth
moved back to Minneapolis from Portland. Beth needed a
roommate, and so did I.

Beth's parents and my parents were long-standing friends.
They enjoyed a weekly doubles tennis game, jointly owned a
sailboat, and had planned outings with all of us kids when we
were growing up. I was also close to Beth's sister Sheila and spent
a lot of time at their home. They had the go-to place, complete
with a swimming pool and pinball machine. As a bonus, their
pantry was always overflowing with sugary cereal (my dad had
banned the sweet stuff from our lives after he read *Sugar Blues*).

Beth and Sheila's dad, with his feisty and entertaining Irish
ways, made me feel more than welcome at their home, as he
boisterously insisted, "Jenny—scoop a bigger helping of those
bloody Lucky Charms!"

After school in ninth grade, Beth and I worked together at
the local dry cleaners. We loved pushing the button that spun
the customers' clean clothes around the clanking metal rack and
swiping credit cards through the old-fashioned carbon paper
imprint machine. With undeveloped professionalism, we giggled
inappropriately every time Mr. Hardon, a regular, said his name
to claim his clothes.

One time, Beth's extra vigorous laughter resulted in her wet-
ting her pants. Not to worry. We spun the clean clothes around

on the loud oval loop until we found a pair she could wear for the rest of the day. (Luckily, the customer who owned those pants didn't come back for pickup until after they had been dry-cleaned a second time.) Beth and I somehow transformed our job from ho-hum to hilarious.

Our apartment hunt began. We found an enchanting one near Lake of the Isles and scooped it up. An alley ran behind the building, and we each snagged an assigned parking spot by the back entrance. A park with trees flanked the alley, where a bounty of leaves showcased the colorful transition to fall.

Built in the early 1900s, the windows in our apartment invited sunlight to flood the space. Compact and complete, our place featured a kitchen, dining area, living room, and two bedrooms. Creamy plaster archways delineated the gathering area from the dining room. Glass corner cabinets, skinny-planked oak floors, and a cheerful ambiance completed the charm.

I'd started sessions with an acupuncturist named Judith, and she'd softened the walls of her treatment room with pale pink paint. Relaxation hugged me in that space, as she'd intended. She'd chosen pink for its properties of inducing peace and calm. Those walls inspired me to paint my apartment bedroom the same color (with the hesitant approval of my landlord). Pink did the trick. My color for calm.

I also cobbled together a richly detailed floral rug, a traditional French baker's rack, and cozy, dive-into-me bedding, all deeply discounted and perfect. I felt tucked in here, like real life was underway. Real life included ongoing dialysis three times a week, but I became accustomed to my routine. Up. Nausea. Dry heaves. Carry on. Clinic one day. Work the next. Fun with Beth. Peace with pink.

That crazy thirst, however, was killing me. Imagine your worst hangover. Your mouth is so dry your tongue sticks to the roof. You crave an enormous glass of ice water. Now imagine that all day long, every day. Yep. That's pretty much what it felt like.

One Saturday afternoon, my mom called. "Do you want to go to a movie?"

"*Steel Magnolias?*" I asked. This movie's story revolves around a group of six women who share friendship and hardship in a small southern Louisiana town. Julia Roberts plays a young woman named Shelby, who has kidney failure and requires dialysis. Her mom (played by Sally Field) donates her kidney.

"It's a dramatic comedy. Let's go laugh," Mom said.

Popcorn in hand, Mom and I sat in our bucket-style chairs and planted our shoes on the sticky floor. Aside from the witty banter in a hair salon, the movie felt like an exaggerated representation of our lives. The concerned mom steeped in worry about her stubborn daughter. The daughter who thought nothing horrible would happen to her.

I'd never seen a movie that depicted a young woman on dialysis, so it held my attention, especially when they discussed Shelby's fistula. Dolly Parton's character said it looked like Shelby had been driving nails into her arm. Check. Fistula confusion. *Cool, I've got that arm too, Shelby.*

I settled in. *These are my movie people.* The don't-stop-me-from-living daughter with her proclamation, stuck in movie lore as a signature line, "I would rather have thirty minutes of wonderful than a lifetime of nothing special." *I like that. Way to say it, Shelby. I want a wonderful life too.*

It all was fine until Shelby rejects her mom's kidney, goes into a coma, and dies. That part wasn't a real knee-slapper for us. Then Sally Field, nominated for a Golden Globe for her performance, unleashes her grief at a cemetery, crying in fits as she screams, "I want to know why!"

My insides tightened as I saw my mom in that Sally Field character, and I didn't want to think of her bellowing in pain at a cemetery on my behalf. I held back tears as I chanted to myself, *It's not real, it's a movie, these are highly paid actors, Julia and Sally are fine, get a grip.* Later, I would learn more about the sadness my mom hid behind closed doors while she cheered me on.

Soon after, my friend Amy saw the movie and said with exuberance, "Wow . . . *Steel Magnolias* is just like your life!"

"I hope not," I replied, grimacing.

"Oh my God, no, no, I just mean the dialysis part," she retorted, her face dropping as she leaned in to squeeze my arm, "not the end!"

"It's okay! Of course I didn't think you were talking about the end." I eased her worry and smiled. I knew what she meant. (Although I'd secretly hoped she thought I was the spitting image of Julia Roberts . . . a girl can dream.) Years later, Amy and I still laugh about that *Steel Magnolias* comment. Because isn't everything better when you laugh?

36

Upside Down

ONE AFTERNOON AT DIALYSIS, SEEMINGLY LIKE ANY OTHER, I arrived and sat in my chair. The air was still. Sue came over and sat down. Her face lacked her usual openness and serene expression. Her lips held straight at the edges.

"What is it?" I asked. I felt the familiar constriction in my throat that signals fear.

"We have some sad news," Sue said, looking solemnly into my eyes. "Tom died last night."

"Tom? Young Tom! What? How?" My body flinched forward as if zapped by an electric charge. I became simultaneously alert and confused from disbelief.

"He had a brain aneurysm and died. A friend found him last night at home, collapsed. He'd already gone." She placed her hand on my knee.

I knew Tom in a medically familiar way; he wasn't my friend per se, more like that rare coworker who encouraged my positivity while he helped me stay alive. That's all. I fought back tears, but they fell anyway.

"I can't believe it," I said.

"None of us can believe it. I have a card for all of you to sign. We will give it to Tom's family." It seemed important to present a card to Tom's family from the people Tom helped every day with his efficiency, compassion, and skills. Did his family and friends have any inkling of what Tom meant to us in the dialysis unit?

How could they really know how his skills made him the home-coming king of our posse? The people in his life should get a glimpse of how much we appreciated what he did and who he was.

Did they know Tom eased Olga's anxiety about needles and soothed her concerns? Did they know Tom righted my blood pressure when I crashed? He was strong and capable—the paragon of perfect health. Shouldn't it have been one of us? It seemed upside down. How unpredictable that eighty-something Olga would outlive thirty-something Tom. I thought about Tom's loved ones who might scream, "I want to know why!"

I wanted to know why. There was no answer.

Tom's death clarified that life isn't lived in degrees. Life is as absolute as pregnancy (and taxes). Dialysis be damned. I was every bit as alive today as Tom had been yesterday. I closed my eyes and prayed that Tom felt he'd had thirty minutes of won-derful in his brief life.

I remembered Elliott's suggestion that we would die young. No one could proclaim to know that I would die young, or someone else would live long. There wasn't a prewritten man-uscript. I ruminated and tried to make sense of the senseless. I realized that age-old question is faulty: Is the glass half-full or half-empty? It assumes the most critical of things—you have a glass. The glass is life. It's everything.

In the wake of Tom's death, life seemed fleeting, temporary, and vital. As I felt the chair solidly supporting me and saw the grief written on the surrounding faces, I took a deep breath and realized my life's uncertainty was not unique. *Life is short. I'm here now. I want to make it matter.*

PART THREE

———

RECEIVING

"It is better to light a candle than to curse the darkness."

—Chinese proverb

37

The Call

AFTER A YEAR AND A HALF ON THE TRANSPLANT LIST, I'D settled into a rhythm, but Tom's death shook me into a new urgency for forward momentum. So I decided that instead of holding steady and waiting for more of my life to begin, I'd chase my dreams. I decided to pursue a master's degree in business at the University of St. Thomas in St. Paul. *Learn. Do. More.*

The first step was to complete the GMATs for my application. Unfortunately, I woke up intensely nauseated on the morning of the exam. I threw up on the way and gave myself props for being prepared with a paper bag.

I plopped in a room filled with bright and eager young faces. Lots of number two pencils at the ready. With a foggy head and rumbling stomach, I slogged through the many questions. I'd made a big mistake. There was no way I would score well on this test. And if I failed, I would ruin everything. All I could think about was how much I hoped I wouldn't toss my toast on the woman sitting in the seat in front of me.

Despite my foggy brain, my test results were good enough, and I completed my application to the program. I received a letter in the mail shortly afterward. I tore it open. Luckily, thankfully, wonderfully, I was accepted.

Unfortunately, as I read further, there was a significant glitch in the acceptance. This business program (to teach me more about business, obviously) required that I gain *more* experience with business first. My acceptance was deferred until I obtained six months of additional time on the job.

Six months felt like an eternity. Wait, wait, wait while a machine cleaned my blood, wait for a transplant, wait for a future to materialize, now this—wait to get my MBA? No! I threw an embarrassing private tantrum, sobbing in fits, while I felt sure my life was forever in neutral.

My dad tried to get me to appreciate that I was, in fact, *accepted* to this program. Despite his attempts to soothe me with his Carnegie wisdom, I wanted to accelerate while outside forces slammed on the brakes.

December blasted in with frigid Minnesota temperatures and covered us in blankets of snow. Quick jogs to a cold car, a hunched posture over the steering wheel until the heat kicked in, short days, long nights, and another birthday. My twenty-fifth. Living with Beth. Still on dialysis.

I wanted something good to happen *now*—I needed to move forward. My energy waned as the light left the skies. I tried to conjure my happiness about being alive, about making the moments matter and taking stock in my lucky list. But lethargy was gaining the upper hand. I felt so tired.

A few months later, it was the beginning of March, that no-season month that bridges the drab winter with the renewal of spring. The snow melted back into the earth, but nothing was in bloom. The lawns were wet with flattened, dormant grass, and the roads looked dirty. The sky offered an unfriendly shade that straddled gray and blue. I repeatedly visualized a transplant—the critical key that would open the door to my better life. Yet it seemed it would never happen.

And then it happened.

It HAPPENED!

A doctor from the University of Minnesota Medical Center reached me by phone at my parents' home. After I'd carried the buzzer so dutifully, it never buzzed. But I heard the doctor say these magic words: "A kidney is available for you." He asked if I could get to the hospital right away. I became jittery, and my stomach did somersaults.

The first Minnesota kidney transplant took place at the University of Minnesota, and their program is one of the oldest and most reputable in the country. In 1982, Dr. John Najarian and the department of surgery received national attention by transplanting a liver into an eleven-month-old girl, Jamie Fiske. This baby girl's life-saving surgery raised national awareness around organ donation.

In 1984, Congress passed the National Organ Transplant Act, which established a computer-generated organ matching system. In 1986, Congress directed federal funds to UNOS. And in March 1990, I jumped into a car with my mom and headed to the University of Minnesota hospital for a new kidney.

38

Light and Dark

THE MOMENT I'D BEEN WAITING FOR ALL THESE MONTHS had arrived! On the one hand, my sole focus had revolved around the upcoming rewards of this transplant, and now it was upon me. On the other hand, I worried about the surgery and the possibility of an unfavorable outcome. What if it didn't work? I swiftly pushed these thoughts aside. I kept reminding myself: *You don't have to do anything—just go to sleep and wake up.*

I saw layers of emotion in my mom's expression, like multiple coats of varnish comprising fear, excitement, and exhaustion. This was *our* call. We shared this illness nightmare, and it was about to end. We shared this transplant dream, and it was about to come true.

I remember a tight hug from Steve. He called Dad. I threw things in a bag, and my mom and I were on our way to the hospital.

The details are a blur. We arrived at the hospital and went through the required pre-surgery steps, but when I try to piece all those steps back together, I can't remember when my dad and Steve arrived. I know they were there. I can't remember what any of the nurses or doctors said. My memory-replay consists of the phone call, drive, prep, IV, and sleep. Approximately four hours after surgery began, I opened my eyes with a new kidney.

My memory sharpens after I woke up because the pain jolted me. The first thing I said through the fog of my medication stupor was, "Nobody told me it would hurt!" It seems obvious—

doesn't everyone realize major surgery hurts? Yet I'd never focused on that part until it was real. An ache radiated from my midsection like a burning fire.

Nurses shouted at me in the recovery room, "Jennifer, can you hear me? Are you awake? Your kidney started to make urine on the table." *My kidney is making urine! How fantastic!*

"On a scale of one to ten, how much does it hurt?"

"A lot!"

I saw faces and bright lights and disassociated from my surroundings, like a dream. I drifted in and out while talking heads hovered over my face.

Nurses pumped morphine into the IV lines, and I faded back into a blurry land with soft edges. Time passed. Soon, I was back in a hospital room, and a team of nurses placed a plastic board under me and slipped me into the bed. I slid over like a fried egg out of a nonstick pan. "You guys have skills," I managed.

Dad and Steve looked scared I might break when I slid over. But Mom was shining. The room looked like many others I'd seen. Flimsy sheets and a worthless paper-thin blanket covered me. I shivered. The clicking of the saline IV sounded to my right, oxygen tubes plugged into my nose, and my midsection radiated that intense sensation from the staples that closed the skin above my new kidney. As my nostrils flared from the amalgamated smells of disinfectant and plastic tubing, nurses encouraged my kidney's good work.

"You're producing a lot of urine. That kidney is happy," the charge nurse said.

"I've been waiting a long time to pee again," I said. Everyone laughed. A laugh as a release, because let's face it, peeing is not that funny. But this normal body function was so welcome, we all had to smile.

I wafted in and out for a while as the anesthesia cleared from my system. Mom, Dad, and Steve hung around, leaving at times to hit the cafeteria and stretch their legs in the halls. Mom fielded the ringing phone and arranged the bouquets of get-well balloons that gobbled up space in the small room. Helium-filled, Mylar messages of thoughtfulness. (The transplant floor didn't allow flowers to avoid the possibility of fungal infections.)

When a nurse insisted that I get out of bed for a little stroll with my IV pole, I thought she was the devil in disguise. There seemed to be no way in hell I'd move.

"I know it sounds hard, but you've got to do a little one," she said. I complied and walked gingerly. Thank goodness for those painkillers. By day two, I was walking well. Slowly. Surely. I called Beth, Lisa, Rae, cousins, other friends. I wanted to talk to everybody.

A team of doctors and residents came marching into my room to examine my incision. As I lifted my hospital gown to expose the fresh scar, the group stood over me and stared quietly, like they were viewing the Mona Lisa. After an awkward pause, the chief resident said, "That's truly lovely." I admired that they took pride in their work. "Behold the beauty, fellows," I said with a big grin, and we all laughed.

They positioned the kidney on the right side of my lower abdomen, and the scar resembled the shape of a boomerang. My original kidneys (in the back) stayed in place. This is typical.

The combination of air and anesthesia irritated my stomach, so I couldn't eat. But fluids were welcome. Hospital staff delivered trays loaded with generous cups of coffee, orange juice, cranberry juice, and Styrofoam pitchers brimming with ice water. It was all mine to enjoy, an unlimited extravaganza of beverages. I'd been thirsty for a year and eight months. Downing those fluids felt like heaven.

Dad walked in as I received my morning tray filled with assorted beverages. "Do you ever want to drink everything in sight?" I asked enthusiastically.

"Not really," he replied, and I remembered, *Oh yeah, that's just me.* He set a cappuccino on my tray—our traditional morning visit. "Thanks, Dad." I drank it down. Best ever. Before he left for work, he paused at the foot of my bed and squeezed my feet, imparting a positive transfer of energy. Our routine.

So it worked. All that focus on good energy paid off.

When I was ready to introduce food, potassium was unrestricted. I'd been dreaming of baked potatoes, tomato sauce, bananas, beans, avocados, yogurt, chocolate, and an endless list of things I couldn't eat before. *It really happened. I really, truly got a kidney!* My spirits soared. Granted, powerful painkillers jacked me up, along with a heavy hit of manic-inducing steroids. Even so, I'd crossed a finish line after a grueling race and achieved my goal. Now everything would be okay.

The transplant team shared little information about my donor. I learned he was a seventeen-year-old young man who'd suffered a car accident in southern Minnesota. I prayed for his grieving family and friends and struggled to reconcile their loss with my gain. It confused me that my future was linked to my donor's loss of life. But I vowed to cherish my donor's benevolence as I carried his kidney forward into the world.

The intersection of life and death were heady subjects for me at twenty-five, and I was immersed in Life Is Complicated 101. I'd revisit this subject again and again in the years to come. How death shapes life, and vice versa. How the contrast of light informs dark. How noise intrudes upon silence. How spring cuts into winter, flowers bloom, trees become green, and those green leaves undergo a colorful metamorphosis, fall away, and eventually the process starts over again.

In the middle of day three, something wasn't right. My urine output slowed down, way down, and the skin around my eyes became swollen. The feeling was devastatingly familiar.

One of the rounding residents came into my room. I propped myself up in bed and told him my concerns. "My urine output has fallen off," I explained, my voice high and tight, "and my eyes are getting puffier." I touched the area under my right eye with my index finger.

"That's not unusual," he said. "We're giving you a lot of medications that can cause swelling. It's helpful to have extra fluid on board to ensure the kidney is well flushed."

I didn't believe him; I knew something was wrong. The shift seemed too sudden.

I summoned Dr. Brown the next day. He listened. "I'll check your urine for protein," he said. He seemed equally scared. If detected, protein would show the unthinkable—FSGS was already at work and causing destructive inflammation.

Sure enough, on day four, the test revealed protein in my urine. Ten insidious, obnoxious, destructive, devastating grams.

Dr. Brown said he wanted to perform a biopsy to confirm his suspicion. Another goddamn biopsy! He wanted to poke holes in my brand-new kidney. It was so unfathomable, so horrible. There was only one thing I could do. As if I had a remote to flip off the thoughts in my mind, I shut off my pain. I didn't want to watch this show anymore. So I made the screen go black.

But later, Dr. Brown walked into my hospital room with sad eyes and said the biopsy confirmed our fears. "Your disease has recurred." He pumped his fist in the air, raised his usually calm voice, and exclaimed, "I did NOT WANT you to have a RE-CURRENCE!"

My gut lurched. He said it was always a possibility, but it doesn't happen often. I have since read it occurs in about 30 percent of FSGS cases. *Did I know this? Did we talk about it?* If we had, I didn't remember, and I was woefully unprepared for this outcome. I had no mental plan B. This transplant was supposed to be the train ride to my future. Where could I go without it?

The dream of returning to Seattle, restored and ready to pick up where I'd left off, evaporated. The dream of ditching the life of compromised kidney function and rebuilding it with normalcy vanished. Nothing in my life had ever felt so utterly beyond my control, because before this recurrence, I'd believed that I could muster *some* control. Through patience, hope, and positive visualizations, I'd reach the promised land. I really believed that. Every fiber of my mental and emotional powers wanted that to be true. I believed in love, medicine, and miracles.

My dreams sank. Would I sink?

Dr. Brown discussed medication options to minimize or slow the progression of this stubborn disease so I could keep the kidney as long as possible. A nurse wheeled me to a classroom on a lower floor, and I learned how to care for my new transplant. Daily medications. Exactly as prescribed. At the right time. In the proper dose.

On the plus side, these medications lower the immune system to help prevent rejection, and on the downside, they lessen resistance to bacterial and viral infections. This made certain things more important. Stay away from sick people. Wash hands frequently. Carry hand sanitizer. Eat healthy foods. Exercise. Start with lab visits three times a week. Show up for regular clinic appointments.

My nurse gave me a manual, like instructions for a new car, a maintenance guide for my new kidney. I could do this. Taking medications on time, no problem. Eating healthy foods and managing all the details, I was a pro. But what I couldn't do—no matter how much I wanted to—was eradicate that autoimmunity, that f**king FSGS. *What now?*

39.

Dinner Pass

ON THE EVENING OF MY FOURTH DAY, I RECEIVED A dinner pass to break away from hospital food. I sat at the table where I'd had so many family meals growing up, elevated my legs on the nearby chair, and rearranged the sautéed chicken around the plate. The smells unsettled my stomach, and my incision felt tender.

If only I could rewind to that moment right after I received the kidney when we jammed into that balloon-filled hospital room with happiness and laughed about pee jokes. The energy of that space had been effusive before FSGS showed up again. If only I could return to the belief that this transplant would fix me, and everything would be okay.

My mom set the table with pretty place mats and her best china. We were celebrating, sort of. I have forgotten whatever conversation took place at that table, but I remember looking at my mom and dad together, as husband and wife, as parents, as a team. They'd been married for about thirty years. They were together as my dad built his business and my mom taught school. They were together for new apartments, houses, and babies. They enjoyed good health. The dinners my cherished parents shared, in their solidly built home, with their unremarkable, everyday moments, struck me as the sum of everything wonderful. A life shared.

I felt like I was falling into a bottomless hole. *Is this possible?*

Can a body keep falling, falling, falling, and never hit the ground? I ached with impossibility.

Dear Universe: I want to give up.

Dr. Brown discharged me the next day. I retreated into my parents' home on Westwood before I returned to my apartment. The week was a blur of resting, recovery, and processing what it would mean that FSGS was still circulating in my system.

I didn't know long this kidney would last. Six months? Six years? Would the FSGS progress rapidly or slowly? How well would the autoimmune medications that prevent rejection slow autoimmune deterioration? Would I forever be measuring everything either against the progression of time or waiting for time to pass?

All the while, friends and family were calling and sending beautiful cards and well wishes for my long-awaited transplant. Did I deserve their positive attention? I had messed this up with recurrence. Was I healthy or not? I didn't know where I had landed on the heal or fail score. I felt ashamed that my body did not take delivery of this gift perfectly. Recurrence rattled my belief in an abundant universe.

Before my transplant, as my kidneys failed, Lasix (the water pill) had no longer worked. But now, because my new kidney worked, Lasix effectively flushed extra fluid. I could drink again and wasn't dreaming about ice water. And the medications to protect against rejection might also slow the escalation of proteinuria, so there was hope there.

Rejection and recurrence were two different things. Rejection is the dreaded reaction when the body recognizes the new kidney isn't your own. When this happens, the immune system attacks the organ like an unwelcome intruder. Good news: No rejection. Bad news: My FSGS planned to hang around. Its nasty mission focused on scarring the filtering units inside my new kidney.

Dr. Brown's mission was to calm my immune system to lessen the severity of the FSGS attack. Hope for the best. And off I would go.

Pills, pills, and more pills. My new kidney required a boatload, some of which necessitated doses precisely twelve hours apart. Swallowing small burrito–sized capsules. Holding my nose for the medication that smelled like skunk spray. It overwhelmed me. I entertained random thoughts (like I could never be on the show *Survivor* unless the producers let me bring my meds and check my labs). Random because I had absolutely no interest in being on *Survivor*. Then I considered all the things I did daily— brush my teeth, take a shower, breathe. If someone told me I had to brush my teeth two times a day for the rest of my life, that might sound like a big deal too.

Daily meds. Just do it.

After about a week, I went back to my apartment. Beth cheered me on as I filled my morning mug full of coffee. "You're having a lot of ounces, Jenny," she said with a big smile.

"A lot more than three." It was one of those little things that felt huge.

And so many other things were better. I didn't need to go to a clinic anymore for treatments. I ate things that were off-limits before the surgery because I had a working kidney, for now. Hello chocolate, bananas, potatoes, pizza, and the occasional salty soup.

Most importantly, at the top of my mind was the tragedy that a young person had died, and his family suffered an unspeakable loss. His family honored his wishes to be a donor, and I was the beneficiary of this unselfish, ultimate act of kindness. I owed it to that family to live the best life I could with their gift.

Dear Universe: Me again. I'm not giving up.

40

Placebo

INITIALLY, WHEN THIS KIDNEY MESS BEGAN, FINGERS pointed in all directions. Perhaps the wood floor finish in the Queen Anne apartment I'd shared with Lisa was toxic to my system. Maybe mercury contaminated the sushi Lisa and I had eaten. Perhaps the ibuprofen I took for headaches inflamed my kidneys. (This theory spurred a team of lawyers to research complications of ibuprofen, but the causal link was weak.) I sleuthed like a bumbling Inspector Clouseau ticking through a potpourri of unrelated factors to pinpoint the cause of my mysterious demise.

Despite attempts to attach blame somewhere, culpability never found an appropriate home. The doctors' consensus was *we might never know what caused this.* Eventually, theories faded into small specks in the rearview mirror.

Dr. Brown started me on new medications to manage the proteinuria and told me to consider a transplant as a vacation from dialysis. Because it wouldn't last forever. He advised me to follow the low-protein/low-fat diet to prolong my kidney's function. And once again, I set out to master the concept of food as medicine.

I voraciously read a book about the pharmaceutical properties of food and learned that the omega-3 fats in tuna were beneficial to slow inflammation. Mustard supposedly hindered inflammation too—I made tuna and mustard my mission.

I also drank apple cider vinegar diluted in water, consumed asparagus, artichokes, watermelon—anything I read about that could improve my health became part of my routine. Would a tuna/mustard/apple cider vinegar cocktail flip a miraculous cellular switch and turn off the autoimmune assault?

My habits proved annoying for some of my friends, especially Ned, whose family cabin in northern Minnesota became our favorite summer retreat. The summer after my transplant, Rachael and Mike, Amy and Ned, Suzanne, Liz, Carrie, and I headed "up north," as we say in Minnesota. I tossed the requisites in a duffel bag—shorts and T-shirts for hot days, cozy sweatshirts for chilly nights, cans of tuna, and a squeeze bottle of mustard.

I fumbled around in the small kitchen one evening and twisted a can of albacore with a handheld opener. I had a self-prescribed daily tuna quota to meet. Amy startled me when she popped around the corner. I dropped the can, and watery chunks fell onto the wide-gapped wood floorboards.

"You scared me. I'm so sorry!" I said, feeling like a complete klutz. A klutz with tuna, no less, and the smell, you can imagine, was pungent. Amy helped me clean it up, but the aromatic evidence lingered in the air. Later, I overheard Ned say to Amy, "What the hell does she need tuna for again?" I cringed.

Whether these food routines were effective or would act as placebos, they gave me a sense of control. The "placebo effect" is a remarkable phenomenon. Throughout the ages, a belief in healing, even when there is no medicine involved, can be transformative. Revival meetings with a miraculous touch, Lourdes holy water, chants, ceremonies, and medicine lodges: there are many routes and rituals intended to spark a powerful healing connection between our brains and bodies.

A captivating case, referenced in *Love, Medicine, and Miracles*, sheds light on the placebo effect with the story of Mr. Wright. In the mid-1950s, he was dying from cancer in his lymph nodes. Bedridden and hardly breathing, he learned of a new anticancer drug called krebiozen. Feeling optimistic, Mr. Wright received his first injection. He experienced immediate improvement. Three days later, he was on his feet and joking with the nurses. Ten days later, he went home. But surprisingly, none of the other krebiozen-treated lymphoma patients got better.

But there's more to the story. About two months later, Mr. Wright read conflicting news reports about krebiozen's effectiveness. He lost faith and suffered an almost immediate relapse. So his psychologist, Bruno Klopfer, told him this big white lie— an improved, doubly effective product was arriving the next day.

That reinvigorated Wright's hope, and he received the double-strength injection. And he improved again! His tumors shrank, and the fluid in his chest disappeared. Except the "medicine" he'd received was only fresh water. He continued to maintain his health with the water treatments until he read another report that krebiozen was ineffective for cancer treatment. His hope vanished, and he died soon after.

The power of his placebo response underscores the intricate link between the body and the mind. If my brain believed that tuna and affirmations improved my condition, so be it. My food choices and visualizations were tools in my body-mind toolbox.

Despite the tuna mishap, the weekend was lovely. My worry over Ned's wrinkled nose dissipated when we hiked through the evergreen forest. Tuna wasn't on anyone's mind as we sat by rushing water and watched it stream over jagged rocks near Lake Superior. And a sense of peace settled in as I absorbed the nature that surrounded us.

Unlike a room I want to rearrange, a paint shade I want to tweak, a jagged scar I want to smooth, or cellular changes I wish for my body, the trees and falling water required no revisions. I never pondered the size of a rock or the bend of a branch. I freed my mind from incessant internal and external editing. How restful is that?

Looking back, I realize I spent every day striving and struggling to control my life somehow. But when surrounded by the natural beauty of Lake Superior, I briefly let myself be.

We roasted marshmallows and told stories under blankets in the big log-walled gathering space. Amy served up bootlegs, her special recipe, as we devoured a big mess of food, including rice, beans, and a variety of tacos.

The 1990s began, ushering in chokers, one-strap undone overalls, and Jennifer Aniston/Courteney Cox–inspired wardrobes. Not to mention the Kurt Cobain–style flannels, and clunky Doc Marten boots paired with light floral skirts. All the rage. Nelson Mandela was released after twenty-seven years in a South African prison, and wrecking cranes tore down the Berlin Wall. I wanted to make it a winning decade.

This cabin getaway reminded me of summer days when my friends and I were in sixth grade and floated down the Apple River in inner tubes. Swimsuits on, lying back, our legs dangling over the edge of the black rubber donut, the current moved us along. We didn't hold on to the banks or resist the water's direction. I longed for that peaceful relaxation more often. And I was beginning to understand that going with the flow only happens when you allow yourself to let go.

41.

Solo

MONTHS PASSED, AND MY ROOMMATE, BETH, ACCEPTED a job opportunity in China. So I found a one-bedroom apartment in a turn-of-the-century brick building, ideally situated off a grass parkway that bridged two Minneapolis lakes. I enlisted help from some big-muscled guys who worked at my dad's company along with a rental moving van. With a charcoal love seat under attack by decorative pillows, a poster of lasagna sketched like an architectural cross section, and two plants I hoped to keep alive, I created a place that felt like home.

And this was a significant realization. Minneapolis had become my home now. I lived in the right place. I did not take it lightly, living solo in my apartment, working at an engaging job, freely drinking ice water without measuring the ounces, and sporting stronger muscles. When I laid my head on my pillow at night and burrowed under my floral duvet, I took stock of all the goodness. I enlisted gratitude, my go-to buddy, and made a point of focusing on the positive things in my life.

And work was one. Work gave me a sense of purpose and legitimized my status as a productive taxpayer. Unencumbered by treatment three times a week, having a full-time position was heaven. My responsibilities continued to grow, and I began to work directly with clients to manage the preconstruction coordination of design, specifications, and contracts.

Stubborn autoimmunity be damned—it didn't outweigh the

other things I had. I didn't allow it to do that anymore. Because I strived to embrace the wise words of philosopher Joseph Campbell: "We must let go of the life we have planned, so as to lead the one that is waiting for us."

One afternoon, I received a call from one of Dr. Brown's nurses, Tommy. She asked if I'd share my outlook with a man who'd received a recent FSGS diagnosis. Flattered that Tommy thought my story might help him, I said yes.

Robert, the CEO of a large local company, was a busy family man with a heavy load of responsibility. He carved out time to make a lunch reservation at a swanky downtown restaurant. With haunting blue eyes, he shared his story and his doctor's treatment plan. We ordered salads and iced tea, and I noticed his pale skin contrasted with his well-tailored dark suit. Anemia, I figured. Through osmosis between me and my kidney doctors, I fancied myself a hack diagnostician.

Robert embodied the dual vibe of a powerful businessman and a gentle soul. So it was easy to talk to him, despite our twenty-year age gap. I shared my belief in lucky lists and the bright side. He thanked me for the visit and said he had gained hope. When we parted, I told him to call me anytime if he needed someone to confide in, complain to, or to offer experience-based empathy.

It was the spring of 1992, two years since I'd received my kidney. Without a cure for FSGS, it became my constant companion. Despite the continued proteinuria causing insidious damage, it was being managed with medications to slow the decline. That long-ago ride home from the Mayo Clinic, when I'd been puffy, emaciated, and scared out of my mind, seemed so long ago. I still feared the inevitable loss of my kidney from this stubborn disease, but being much less immediate, I tucked that fear away.

My brother, Steve, had moved back to Manhattan, much happier, as he began a master's degree program in screenwriting. Graduate school began for me too, and I started business classes on Tuesday/Thursday evenings (after work) and Saturday mornings. I quickly befriended Larry—a self-deprecating, long-faced dog lover who made graduate school bearable.

We frequently studied at his condo, which is where I eventually met Larry's girlfriend, Dawn. A petite, soft-spoken brunette with short, cropped hair, Dawn's doe eyes evoked those of the cartoon character Betty Boop.

After Larry and Dawn decided to take a relationship break, Dawn moved into an open apartment unit one floor down from mine. Larry's loss was my gain. Now I had the best of apartment situations—a place of my own, plus a close friend a few units away. How delightful to be the Mary Tyler Moore to her Rhoda. (I cast myself as Mary, of course, because as the theme song goes, I too wanted to make it after all.)

Dawn and I navigated singlehood together and experienced our fair share of awkward dates. Dawn suffered through a lunch-turned-rollerblading-turned-dinner date from hell, while I went out with a guy who curiously responded to my every statement with an enthusiastic "Jeepers creepers!"

Meanwhile, Lisa and I stayed in touch and compared notes on our lives. She'd started dating a guy named Mike, who'd attended the same college we did. He was a few years ahead of our class, so I didn't know him while we were on campus.

"How's it going with Mike?" I asked.

"Mike's great," Lisa said. "Getting serious, I think." Her voice sounded clear and bright.

A vicarious thrill rushed through me. I could hear her smile and picture her happiness. "Oh my God, Lisa, you're in love with Mike?! That's awesome! And I'm jealous."

"You're jealous because you want to be in love with Mike?" she teased. As I laughed, I couldn't help but wonder about her future. Had she found the one? Lisa's "normal" life became the barometer for mine. I felt somewhat content with my modified "normal"—despite it all, I had an apartment, friends, a job, independence, some dates sprinkled in, and graduate school underway.

And I tried to limit thoughts about my inevitable uncertainty: *How long will this transplant last?* Although knitted into that ambiguity was another clamoring concern. *Was Steve right years ago when he questioned if I'd ever get married? Who signs up for a ticking kidney time bomb?* I inhaled a slow breath. I blew it out through my rounded lips and redirected my fear. *It's okay. Being alone might be the best thing.*

Well, that's what I tried to convince myself, anyway. Expectation management. But if I was being honest, did I really believe being alone would be the best thing?

42

Sunbreak

ONE LAZY SATURDAY AFTERNOON IN MAY, DAWN AND I walked out to sunbathe in the Parkway. Ready for a break, she stood up, grabbed her towel, and said, "Get the story on that guy hitting golf balls for me. He's cute."

I glanced the golfer's way as Dawn retreated inside. He looked up and smiled. After a few minutes, he walked over in his navy swim trunks with a golf club in hand. Brown hair. Friendly eyes. Muscles in a trim body. He introduced himself as Dirk Miller. And within a short time, he covered many topics—his family, his friends, his profession (an eating disorder specialist working on his PhD at the University of Minnesota).

"Do you golf?" he asked.

"No."

"Let me show you." He stood behind me, positioned the club in front, and moved my arms in a sample swing. My yellow-and-pink-striped bathing suit exposed me a tad, but that was nothing compared to revealing my prominent fistula as I extended my arms to the club. This Dirk guy didn't say a thing about it, so I assumed that as a medical student specializing in eating disorders he must have encountered fistulas in his education. I breathed deep relief that I didn't have to explain.

After we completed our golf lesson and chat fest, I darted straight to Dawn's apartment.

"What's his deal?" she asked.

I told Dawn all the dirt. Dirk lived in the apartment next

door. He'd grown up in Pennsylvania with his brother and two sisters in a small town southeast of Pittsburgh. He was a fanatical Steelers fan, loved to golf—did I mention he was a fanatical Steelers fan? (it's worth repeating)—had his PhD in process, and was our neighbor.

"Wow, you really got a lot of background," she said. She handed me a glass of water, and we flopped on her sofa.

"He spilled." I patted myself on the back for all the intel I'd gathered for her. Sure, he'd saddled up behind me to demonstrate a golf move, but I didn't feel a spark. This was a mission to find a new boyfriend for Dawn, not me.

The next day in the lobby of our apartment, Dawn saw Dirk buzzing my apartment's doorbell. He turned to her and said, "I was going to ask Jennifer out for dinner." When she told him I wasn't home, he continued (awkwardly and slightly embarrassed, he confessed later), "Well . . . do you want to go out for dinner?" Dawn told him she couldn't make it, but she'd mention to me he'd stopped by.

My reaction when Dawn told me about it later that night was: "That's sweet. Dirk is looking for new friends."

"Why do you assume he wants to be friends?" she asked, her eyebrows lifted.

"Why do you assume not?" I asked. "Some guys want female friends. We don't know." I wasn't jumping to her conclusions.

She shot me a stern glance and shook her head from side to side. Then she slowly said as if she was teaching a naive child a valuable lesson, "Listen, Jennifer—no straight single guy will *ever* want to be your friend." We launched into a *When Harry Met Sally* debate. Dawn sided with Harry, who claimed that men and women couldn't be friends without complicated feelings clouding the picture. I (Sally) felt certain men and women could just be buddies.

I laughed during our breezy conversations about guys, but underneath, I didn't see myself the way Dawn saw me. I classified myself as better friend material than girlfriend material. Or at least better suited for a casual relationship versus one with direction. I was imperfect and damaged. With persistent autoimmunity permeating my thoughts, I didn't score myself high on the lovability/romance scale.

The next day, the noise from the round bell mounted by my door startled me. "Hi," I said as I opened the door, surprised to see Dirk so soon. My heart sped up. "That buzzer is so loud. Does your apartment have those doohickeys too?" I stepped aside to let him in.

A perplexed grin made his eyes sparkle. "I don't know what you're talking about . . . but I'm sure I don't have any doohickeys." Pointing to the wall-mounted bells, I laughed at his reaction to my imprecise terminology. "I came to see if you want to grab dinner?" he asked. His eyes moved in all directions to get a glimpse of my apartment. Bonus points. It was tidy.

Was Dawn right? My energy lifted with his invitation. Instead of a lonely make-do-with-what-was-in-the-fridge dinner (Egg Beaters and tomato soup), dinner with Dirk offered more flavor. We walked down Dean Parkway, past the green where we'd met the day before, and stopped at the corner restaurant across from Lake Calhoun. I learned more about him, told him more about me, and felt myself relax.

At the end of the evening, he said, "You have beautiful eyes," and stared right through them. I froze and averted my gaze with sudden shyness. Then a frosty chill ran through me. I looked back toward him, and he held my gaze. I realized that his brown eyes were beautiful too. Okay, I got it—this was the first date with my new "friend" Dirk.

Later that night, I gave Dawn the play-by-play. She scolded

me, "You shouldn't let some stranger buzz their way into your apartment! What if you'd let in a serial killer?" Perhaps she had a point. Although it was only one date, as far as I could tell, Dirk offered no visible clues that he might be a serial killer. (But what did I know about serial killer clues?) I looked into his cocoa-brown eyes, however, and saw a handsome guy with a kind soul.

I figured I'd take the chance.

43

Shouting Secrets

MY SECOND DATE WITH DIRK TOOK PLACE AT A
kitschy restaurant called Chez Bananas in the Minneapolis
Warehouse District. Tucked into a booth with Mr. Potato Head
and a Magic 8 Ball on the tabletop, we enjoyed tropical drinks
and awaited spicy Caribbean meals. Our conversation sparked,
true to form for a new relationship, and I learned about Dirk's
favorite movies. I (patiently) listened to him recite word for
word his memorized lines from *Dirty Harry*:

"I know what you're thinking. 'Did he fire six shots or only
five?' Well, to tell you the truth, in all this excitement I kind of lost
track myself." I started to interrupt, but he kept going, "You've got
to ask yourself one question: 'Do I feel lucky?' Well, do ya, punk?"

"You sweet talker, you, I bet you say that to all the girls."

When I told Steve (an avid movie buff) about my date with
Dirty Harry, he said, "I've got to meet this guy."

On our third date, Dirk and I walked back to our neighborhood restaurant and sat at the same high top by the window.
Perched on a stool, I looked out across the street that separated
us from Lake Calhoun, the same lake where Nick had revealed
his discomfort with my freakishness. As always, bikers, walkers,
and rollerbladers peppered the path that circled the lake. Sailboats
and canoes dotted the water. All these active people beyond the
window displayed life in action. And here I was, on a date with
Dirk, living mine.

But after we crossed the line of my illness, would he lose interest? I tightened up my emotional armor; I didn't want to think ahead and worry he might walk away.

Afterward, we walked around and talked. We dropped into discovery mode. I told him I had an undergraduate business degree from the University of Puget Sound and explained how much I loved the Pacific Northwest. To add extra polish to my credentials, I told him the president at Puget Sound referred to our school as the Harvard of the West.

"That's funny," he said, "because I think the president of Harvard refers to their institution as the Puget Sound of the East." Clever. We walked past the previous apartment I'd lived in with Beth and compared notes on our shared landlord. I heard about his PhD program and told him about my MBA program, but all the while my secret nagged at me. *You've got to tell him.* But I wasn't ready to share it yet. Why add weight to something so light and fun?

I wanted an ordinary life and feared my illness might shut it all down. In this stage of our early flirtations, I appeared normal. And I didn't want to depart from that feeling and face the reckoning to come—his evaluation of my true self. He hadn't called me a freak. And I didn't want him to.

He reached for my hand, and we kept walking. It surprised me to learn he was thirty-five, eight years older than me. He had been so absorbed in his career, master's degree, and PhD that he hadn't had time to commit to a relationship. At the end of the night, we kissed. Definitely nice, but I planned to take it slow.

For now, if he saw me as dateable, that seemed a better alternative than damaged.

A week later, I flew to Seattle for Lisa and Mike's wedding. It excited me to join the wedding party. As the plane traveled the airspace between the Midwest and the West Coast, I thought of my previous flights on this route: as an eighteen-year-old on the way to college, as a twenty-two-year-old flying home for a biopsy, as a twenty-four-year-old returning to Seattle again as a dialysis patient, back to Minneapolis to await my kidney, and now, happily joining Lisa for her wedding weekend.

Lisa arrived at the airport, and we turned in a circle while we hugged. "Lisa! You're getting married!" I exclaimed.

"I know!" she said, as if she could hardly believe it herself.

"You look amazing," I chimed as I noticed the healthy blush in her flawless skin. "Love looks good on you."

True to her chic style, she selected sleeveless linen dresses for the bridesmaids that fell just above the knee. A simple dress, with the intent (as always) that we could wear it again. (Take a guess if I ever wore it again . . . Has *anyone* ever worn it again?)

She glowed on her wedding day, and her dress transformed her into an ethereal princess. Mike beamed at her and eloquently expressed his love at their reception dinner. The lovefest and a wee bit of wine got to Lisa. As I looked at her, her face broke into a squished-up, overcome-with-emotion cry. I was witnessing her happily-ever-after Kodak moment.

And I couldn't help but daydream about Dirk.

It was lovely and official. My friend Lisa, my once eighteen-year-old college roommate, was moving on, and the world shifted a bit. It had been Lisa and me for so many years in college, where we'd both imagined our future careers, lives, and husbands. It had been Lisa and me for five months in Seattle in two different apartments. It had been Lisa who I called during my ordeal and often ever since. Now it was Lisa and Mike. And it resembled the bittersweet pang after finishing a wonderful

book. In the last chapter, I don't want to leave those characters.
Now I understood one story was over, and a new one would begin.

Back in Minneapolis, Dirk and I enjoyed Korean food at a restaurant in Uptown. His movie references continued.

"You talkin' to me? You talkin' to me? You talkin' to me?"

"I know this one! De Niro. *Taxi Driver*."

Besides learning that Dirk was a fan of movies and open to a variety of cuisines, I found him to be confident, intelligent, and attractive. A connection was underway, so my secret shouted at me. *Tell him! Let him measure your value with accurate information!*

In between forkfuls of seasoned vegetables with chicken and rice—with burning cheeks and sticky palms—I blurted out, "I've got bad kidneys."

"Tell me more," he said, true to the response you'd expect from a psychologist.

"It's an autoimmune thing. I've had a transplant. And I'll need another. I don't know when." I flew my red flags. It was our fourth date, and now he could calculate his interest by knowing one sure thing—my package came with uncertainty.

I studied his expression; it held steady.

"Dessert?" he asked. That wasn't the question I'd expected. We peeled ourselves from the red vinyl booths of the small restaurant and walked out into the Minneapolis summer night. Cooking smells lingered on our clothes.

"How old were you when you first got sick?" he asked as we walked down the street. He slowed his typically fast pace to match mine.

"Twenty-two," I said. "This has been my deal for five years. My illness hit completely out of the blue."

"When I was twenty-two, I hit rock bottom myself," he explained.

"What happened?"

"Let's just say I was a little too enthusiastic about drinking. First, I went through hell, then I went through treatment." He'd obviously said this before, but I liked his honest delivery. He offered a boyish smile. "So I'm sober now." His cards were also on the table. I had suspected as much by the non-alcoholic beer he'd ordered on our first date.

I liked that he was well acquainted with the hidden snipers lurking in life. He implied that maybe we'd both endured difficulties in ways hard to compare, but still, difficulty does not discriminate. Dirk's sobriety had been underway for twelve years, and he was fully comfortable if people around him drank alcohol. He'd accepted that his version of a good life would exist without drinking. And his wisdom on life's challenges seemed unique and refreshing.

Although I wasn't that familiar with AA, I'd later learn that AA principles align with my approach to navigating chronic illness. The best way to avoid being overwhelmed by tomorrow is to take one day at a time. (Maybe Ida wasn't so loony after all.)

"Do you want some ice cream?" he asked. I knew he was an ice cream lover.

"I have another confession," I said. "Brace yourself . . . I'm not a big fan of ice cream." He pondered this critical reveal for a few seconds. The kidney transplant went over pretty well, but I wondered if frozen dessert might be the deal breaker. (At least I'd nailed that De Niro quote.) Finally, he said, "Okay, we can make this work if I eat the ice cream and you drink the alcohol."

"That works for me," I said, and we smiled.

I considered marriage as something reserved for my friends and actresses in Kodak commercials, so I didn't allow that on my radar. My feelings were less complicated than that. I delighted in his companionship and the knowledge that we'd shared our "defects" and the world kept spinning. He reached for my hand. And we walked with the realization that something good was in the air.

44

Exclusive Club

AT WORK, MY DAD SHARED HIS WEALTH OF INFORMATION and was an exemplary teacher. Together, we explained the custom home process to new clients, and I guided them through the series of preconstruction steps. The various selections that made each home unique enthralled me. And since I'd been searching for a sense of home myself, the literal and figurative concept was near and dear to my heart.

I guess it always was. As a young girl, I frequently rearranged my bedroom furniture, eager to explore the renewal in changing compositions. My job ignited this same creative wonder as I teamed closely with not only clients but also interior designers, architects, photographers, and graphic designers. This fabulous job energized my happiness.

My dad had lived in Minnesota his entire life. The son of a grocer, he'd folded into the family business at a young age. He worked with his younger brother, Bob, at the store after school. While my grandma Helen balanced the books, my grandpa Jerry operated the store and tended to every detail, including hand-painting the outdoor signs to advertise the prices per pound of meats and poultry. Brothers Larry and Bob helped with everything from greeting the customers to sweeping the floors to stocking the shelves. Cramer's Food Mart—a family affair.

By the time he was in eighth grade, my dad had connected to his ambition, soaked up the business skills of his father, and strived to emulate the high integrity he'd witnessed while working at the store. He studied history at the University of Minnesota, got a job in mortgage banking, and found his calling in the custom home business. His job involved construction management of luxury homes for clients.

High standards and customers who rightly demanded exceptional service were his specialty. Likability was his strength thanks to his unflappable nature, low-key personality, and straightforward honesty. Being part of a family business was what he knew, so it pleased him that I contributed to the company.

But I didn't see it that way. Not at first.

Dad consistently introduced me as his daughter. I bristled because I wanted him to regard me as a businessperson with a valuable set of skills. In my mind, his introduction reduced me to "she has a chronic illness; there is nowhere else for her to work." But I wanted to stand out for the job I did, not the daughter I was. I often wondered what would have happened if I'd had the chance to complete my Seattle PR internship. After impressing Stacy, and launching into the world, what job would I have landed then?

One day, in frustration, I asked, "Why do you have to tell everybody I'm your daughter?"

As if my words stung him, his face pinched, and he said, "I'm proud you're my daughter, and I want people to know."

The change in his expression made me regret what I'd said. How could I have been half-blind to the value of these precious opportunities? The PR position in Seattle was only valuable because it presented the bottom rung of a career ladder. I'd focused so much on that lost ladder, failing to recognize that Dad had put another in its place.

Initially, both he and I knew a job was imperative for my sense of self-worth and for being "normal." But as it turned out, with my abilities, I climbed the rungs. My business degree and master's degree work were valuable, but he could find those skills in other professionals. Because I did a good job *and* was his daughter, he felt proud. As a people pleaser, what could've been better than simultaneously pleasing both my dad *and* my boss?

I had fallen short on a basic Dale Carnegie lesson: Put yourself in the shoes of another and see things from their point of view. I reconsidered our working arrangement from my dad's perspective, and I got it. Our family connection was something to celebrate, not something to conceal.

From that point forward, I enthusiastically introduced myself as the daughter of Larry Cramer. And I recognize it is a unique distinction, a very exclusive club—because I'm the only lucky girl to boast with pride that Larry Cramer is her dad.

45

Survivors

MY INFATUATION MONTAGE WITH DIRK FEATURED restaurants, movies, baseball games, festivals, art fairs, bike rides, strong coffees, ice creams for Dirk, and drinks for me. I learned Dirk grew up in a modest home on several acres in rural Pennsylvania. His teenage drinking offered him a quick and easy escape from his religious upbringing and small town.

A mess of DWIs, run-ins with the police, and drunken escapades (lively fodder for future AA meetings) led to treatment at twenty-two, bolstered by the insistence of his concerned parents.

Twenty-eight days later, he walked out of rehab and never had a drink again.

I didn't appreciate at first how much strength it must have taken Dirk to abandon alcohol completely at such a young age, because few people in my life had alcohol issues. But I've since learned how rare it is to walk away from addiction as resolutely as Dirk did. No relapses. No victimhood. No self-pity. He impressed me early on, and later, I'd admire him even more when I watched him inspire many others.

Dirk also wrestled in high school, and he felt enormous pressure to make weight, along with his fellow athletes. In many cases, this heightened focus on the scale fostered bulimia. This exposure, coupled with his sister Emily's struggle to overcome anorexia and bulimia (which she did, thank goodness), inspired his public health and psychology degrees. From there, he earned his PhD to specialize in eating disorder treatment.

I noticed how he carried and defined himself; he didn't tell his story with shame. He embraced his struggles and moved confidently in the world. This made him so appealing; he had real-life insights instead of an idealized version of what life should be.

Maybe that's why our relationship came easily. I couldn't articulate it then, but our unique life experiences connected us through something we shared—survival instinct. And my fistula and scar, imperfections that seemed like flashing caution signs to me, were nonexistent barriers to romance for Dirk. Just as his alcohol addiction did not deter my interest.

I should have thought of my scar as a symbol of successful healing and the pursuit of a happy life. And my fistula, as much as I hated it (and hid it), was my valuable in-place access to life if I needed to use it again for dialysis. Dirk clarified these medical souvenirs were not me—scars don't have personalities, make people laugh, or spark playful conversations. Or fall in love.

Was I falling in love? It was going well, but I still held tight to emotional safeguards. *This is fun for now. I'll enjoy this while I have it.* Perhaps I applied Dr. Brown's transplant vacation philosophy to dating Dirk. Or maybe I'd lost the idealism of my younger self since Nick slammed me for being a "freak." I didn't know how long this relationship with Dirk would last, but I'd appreciate every moment while I could. I enjoyed my Cinderella-at-the-ball moment, except I didn't know when the stroke of midnight would come.

One evening, Dirk and I watched *Seinfeld* together, cuddled on my love seat. I stretched my legs over his lap, and he massaged my calves. In an instant, my teeth chattered as an internal blast of cold sent me into shivers. Dirk fetched a thermometer—104 degrees. My fevered eyes seemed to look through thick green glass with fog on the other side.

Dirk immediately called my doctor, the transplant clinic,

and my parents. He insisted on taking me to the hospital. Once there, I begged for hot blanket after hot blanket. The doctors and nurses worked to get my temperature down, so they ignored my pleading and started IV fluids. The continuous drips from the saline bag pumped ice water through my veins.

A bladder infection took hold and spiked my fever. Here was one of those side effects the transplant clinic had warned me about: greater susceptibility to infections. And it swooped in so rapidly—I didn't have symptoms until the shaking began. IV antibiotics to the rescue. Within a few days, the infection was under control.

This hectic night in the emergency room, of all places, was where my mom and dad first met my new boyfriend. One thing became immediately clear to them—Dirk was a caring, take-charge guy. We'd learn later what miracles would come from his make-it-happen nature.

46.

A Leap

AT TWENTY-SEVEN YEARS OLD, I WAS A BUSINESS STUDENT with a cute companion and a full-time job. My kidney also continued doing its full-time job. For now. Dirk and I spent our weekends at his place, powering through the requirements to expand our educations in psychology and business. While he focused laser-like on his dissertation, I buried my nose in MBA textbooks.

A lone dark-green leather sofa, a six-pack of Diet Coke, and a well-used coffee maker comprised his clean, spare interior. His minimalist apartment contrasted with my decorated (chock-full-of-accessories) unit next door. My space featured abundance and strived for a pleasing presentation. His interior had nothing to prove. It was what it was.

By three o'clock in the afternoon, after nonstop studying and writing, my ravenous stomach rumbled. "Don't you want to eat?" I asked. "Let's take a break and grab lunch."

"No. I've got to keep going," he said without looking up from his computer. I left him to write frenetically like Jack from *The Shining*, while I ventured out for sustenance. All work and no food makes Jenny a dull girl.

Dirk immersed himself in his relentless dissertation mission and encouraged his classmates to power through as well. He had an encouraging "joke" at the ready. "Do you know what you call the person with the worst dissertation?" He'd pause for effect, and say, "Doctor."

The point of the joke underscored his drive. His singular "doctor" focus, however, diluted his focus on me. I wondered if my time had come and gone as I sunk with discouragement about his waning attention.

We spent time with another couple, Trish and Joe, friends of Dirk's from college in Indiana. They had recently moved to Minneapolis. Joe knew Dirk inside and out, so he became easy to talk to about my frustrations. "He's not into it anymore," I said.

"You need to give him a little time. He retreats when he has something big on his mind," Joe explained.

"Yeah, well, this dissertation could take a long time, and I'm frustrated," I said. I missed the initial spark, and I didn't understand what had happened to the choice guy I dated. Where did *that* Dirk go? His conversations dried up as he fell into a continuous mode of quiet rumination.

"All I can say is, wait it out, it's not what you think," Joe said, and opened his eyes wide. He held my look for emphasis. I had no idea what kind of excuse he was making for Dirk, but I trusted him. At the same time, I needed to protect myself. Marriage wasn't my focus, but I wanted to enjoy the person with whom I spent my time currency on.

If the relationship energy was fading and affection and love weren't there, I didn't want to hang around. I mentioned none of these thoughts, however, to Dirk. I shared some with Joe and bottled the rest up. Later, I would learn this hold-it-in tendency of mine was emotionally equivalent to overstuffing papers into a file cabinet—eventually, you get a messy overflow.

While I thought our story might end, Joe knew Dirk was merely getting his ducks in a row so he could launch a new beginning.

Finally, Dirk's big day arrived. He presented his final oral examination to the dissertation committee. They unanimously recommended his eligibility to receive his doctoral degree and graduate. As he left, a member of the committee uttered three words that made his hard work (and his overused joke material) worthwhile: "Congratulations, Dr. Miller."

That achievement revived him. The dullness lifted, and he morphed into a hyper, sugared-up kid at a playground. His eyes danced, and his energy became unstoppable. We celebrated over lunch and giddily browsed through downtown shops. Dirk was ebullient as he floated through the afternoon. At the ready with hugs, side squeezes, and kisses for me, Dr. Miller also cranked up his charisma and charmed all the salespeople we encountered.

PhD complete. One duck down.

I didn't realize, however, that I was the next duck.

On a Saturday at the end of October, Dirk and I worked at our respective offices to wrap up loose ends before the next workweek began. He called and asked if I would join him in St. Paul for a bite to eat. I warned him I had on a ripped, oversized green sweatshirt and black workout leggings.

"It doesn't matter," he assured me. "Meet me at my clinic office. We'll go somewhere from here." We shared vibrant moods. I felt his energy through the phone and anticipated a fun night ahead.

From his office, we went to a nearby quaint restaurant called Muffuletta. We sat in bistro chairs at a simple wood table covered in cream linens. "I'm pretty underdressed," I said to him in a whisper as I looked around at the other diners.

"Who cares?" he replied flippantly, and reached for my hands on the table.

"Yeah . . . who cares," I said, unleashing a wild grin. The world beyond us had faded away; it was just Dirk, my ripped sweatshirt, and me.

I don't remember all the specifics of our sparkly exchanges

to follow, but we soared into the intoxicating relationship groove where every tidbit seemed hilarious or deeply meaningful. When our meals arrived, I picked at mine slowly. Nibble. Gab. Nibble. Gab. Dirk had long since finished his meal and fidgeted in his seat.

"Are you done yet?" he asked.

"No."

"Really?"

"Really," I said. I was the slow eater of our duo, and it befuddled him how I could make a meal last. I moved my fork in a slow-motion gesture to tease him.

"Be done already! Put your cutlery down." He was oddly insistent.

It amused me we bantered about my cutlery status. Who talks about cutlery? Finally, I finished, and the server cleared my plate. Soon after, he returned with a flute of champagne and a bounty of red roses. Dirk's eyes sparkled while he suppressed a smile.

"Why did the waiter bring me flowers and champagne?" I asked slowly. A whoosh of confused emotion sucked the air from my lungs, and my giddy smile flattened.

Dirk pulled out a ridiculous plastic bracelet shaped like a diamond ring. After he held it high, he handed it to me across the table. With a grand smile, he said, "Will you marry me?"

What's happening? We had never discussed marriage, so his proposal caught me entirely off guard. I froze, wide-eyed and speechless. The silence blasted.

"What are you thinking right now?" he asked, while his unanswered question hovered in the air between us.

First thoughts: *Did he just ask me to marry him? On Halloween? That fake ring in the form of a bracelet is a joke. Is this whole thing a joke?* Then the seriousness of what he'd presented swarmed me. One side of me held tight to the idea that this relationship was fun, and I deserved fun. And love. Yes, of course, love. The other side fretted over my potential for ongoing medical disasters. This part carried my past trauma—my young self's breach of contract with "normal" life. "What about my health?" I asked in a quiet, cracked tone. My stomach clenched into a knot. *Why is he doing this? He knows all about me.*

Dirk's eyes flooded. "We'll deal with whatever we need to deal with. Together."

The "we" struck me. That small word seemed to defy loneliness in such a big way. I also knew that between his lines delivered with romantic conviction, behind his determined brown eyes, he was hesitant and scared shitless. Maybe we could move forward, hesitant and scared shitless together. He invited me to take a leap with him, uncertainty and all.

The twinkle in Dirk's eyes faded. His face shifted from excitement to complete vulnerability. "You *are* going to say yes, aren't you?" he said, flickers of distress evident in his tone. He radiated tenderness. Pulled from my thoughts, I remembered this moment exposed him too.

But my mind raced ahead and continued to bombard me with fears. *What kind of future is Dirk signing on for? Will I be a drag of a wife? I can't believe he wants to stick it out with me— maybe I do have a future. He's obviously betting on it—that fake ring better be a joke ring. Marriage? Can I do this? Should I take the leap?* I thought back to Tom, the dialysis technician, and his unexpected death. Uncertainty is part of life; best to live it now.

Impulsively, I answered the questions bouncing around my brain—*I will leap.* Suddenly, I envisioned the future I had not allowed myself to entertain. A cascade of images toppled into rapid-fire statements of the obvious.

"We could have a dog!"

"We could have a house!"

"We could have a kid!"

Dirk smiled. "Yes, we could." He remained patient with my proclamations of the obvious, God bless him.

Finally, with a stupid smile spanning my face, I answered the question. "Yes, I will marry you."

47

Burden or Bother

WE WENT BACK TO DIRK'S APARTMENT, GIDDY WITH excitement and teary with emotion. *Engaged* was a magical word, and I couldn't believe it was one I could use in conversation about myself. Engagement is for people who plan for a future.

"You should call your mom and dad," Dirk said. My eyes filled at once, although I was smiling too.

"I need to wait and get myself together," I replied, shaking my head to rattle myself into a more composed state.

"I'll call them." And with that, Dirk dialed their number, got them both on the phone, and said, "Your daughter has accepted my proposal of marriage." He beamed. It sounded so official, like he was making a pronouncement to a royal court. I giggled through tears as he smiled at me. His eyes filled up too.

Because Dirk was signing up to share my life wholly, he researched my illness and educated himself about dialysis and kidney transplantation—medical lifelines we would rely on when my current transplant petered out from autoimmune assaults. We set up a proactive meeting with Dr. Brown to manage expectations. To summarize our visit, Dr. Brown told Dirk, "I think Jennifer's health will be more of a bother than a burden."

It was nice to know I would not be a burden, but I can't say I loved the classification of being a bother. It was hard to remember that we were talking about my stubborn autoimmunity, not me, and it was still a challenge for me to separate the two. Dirk and I would get married in the summer, and the kidney stuff would hang around with us forever.

To save money, we consolidated our side-by-side apartments to live in Dirk's bigger apartment in the months before the wedding. I moved into his building right next door.

Surprising emotions surfaced about leaving my space. My first independent apartment. I felt accomplished; I had a job, paid my rent, owned my car, and made my life work. Now I was saying goodbye to this version of myself and hello to another. Would I lose myself when I folded into a marriage? I figured that couple skills might be like managing chronic uncertainty—you can't predict how it will unfold, so you plunge in and stay upbeat. I would learn later that being married was significantly more complicated than staying upbeat.

Dirk helped me get my stuff together. It was time to bid farewell to my space so I could merge my life with Dirk's. Bags packed, door open, I took a long look at my charming, now empty apartment.

The thin-planked oak wood floors, the plaster archways, the little hexagon bathroom tiles that never seemed clean (no matter how hard I scrubbed them), the tiny kitchen—this place had become my familiar home. As tears wet my eyes, I said goodbye to my single life. I had become fond of her, that Mary Tyler Moore version of myself.

I remembered when I'd asked my mom, years earlier, after illness initially hammered me, "What if I'll always be alone?" I feared the confines of being a nephrotic girl, or "a goddamn nephrotic," as that jackass surgeon had proclaimed. Now I was venturing beyond my single girl identity. But instead of doing it alone, I'd travel through life with my soon-to-be husband.

Dirk put his arm around me, and his squeeze conveyed reassurance. The universe and Dirk were on my side. Maybe it tipped the scales—pumping all those visualizations and abundance into what I wanted to manifest in my life. I nestled further into my fiancé's side. The question I'd asked my mom years earlier about being alone had an answer. I said hello to the next chapter—my life with Dirk.

48

Wonderful World

ON A PERFECT DAY IN JUNE 1994, BILL CLINTON WAS the president, Jackie O graced the cover of *Time*, and Dirk and I got married.

We hired a string quartet that played my favorite traditional folk song, "The Ash Grove." I learned this melody in my sixth-grade choir class. My mom knew it well because I tinkered it constantly on the piano keys in the family room after school in junior high. When the quartet played this song at our wedding, I turned around, smiled at her, and winked.

It had been a year since Lisa's wedding, and now it was Lisa's turn to be my bridesmaid. Rachael (married to Mike) was also a bridesmaid. Beth was my maid of honor, and Dawn (who'd since reunited with and become engaged to Larry) was my personal attendant. Cindy, Susan, and Gillian flew in from Seattle. Ecstatic that so many friends and family joined us to celebrate, and woozy with wonder, I was overjoyed that marriage wasn't just for other people. It was for me too.

Father John Malone, a previous colleague of Dirk's at the counseling center of the University of St. Thomas in St. Paul, presided at our wedding. Father Malone was a funny guy, and his humor often caught people off guard. It certainly did for me when he stated at the beginning of our wedding ceremony in the awe-inspiring volume of the Catholic church, "I thought it would be a cold day in hell when Dirk Miller got married."

Everyone laughed. I fake-laughed. Wedding wisecracker. We said our "I do's" and spilled into a limo—a wedding gift from Dirk's friend Scott. It was a friendly gesture, but Scott, a sucker for a bargain, didn't realize the "classic" limo was an ancient "beauty" without air-conditioning. I leaned forward on the ride to the reception so sweat wouldn't trickle down my backside. Melting makeup and a hot limo were not part of my plan! Yet when Dirk held my hand, I realized if we were in this hot, stuffy limo together, it was darn near close to perfect.

At the reception, three buffet stations featured a variety of entrées (I borrowed this idea from Lisa's wedding), and everything tasted delicious. Flowers filled the room. The invitees were celebratory. The fabulous band played a variety of music that engaged all age groups. And Dirk and I rejoiced.

Even Elvis made an appearance. When I heard someone say they'd spotted Elvis in the building, I didn't realize a terrible Elvis impersonator (in a white polyester suit and ill-fitting black wig) would bomb the reception and sing "Love Me Tender." Another gift from Scott. Remarkably, the guy seemed more like an impersonator *of* a bad Elvis impersonator.

After Elvis left the building, Dirk and I laughed off the unforeseen wedding crasher. And really, the surprise was a fitting start to our marriage because we'd learn that all well-laid plans get punctuated with the unexpected.

My dad and I danced to a modified "Brown Eyed Girl," a tune more up-tempo than he realized, so midway into our routine, with obvious discomfort, he whispered, "How long *is* this song?" I laughed. He wasn't as composed as the Kodak commercial father who had unhinged me years earlier in the Seattle summer house. But I wondered if he similarly reminisced about all the milestones that had unfolded before this day.

Dirk and I danced slowly to "What a Wonderful World."

The lyrics perfectly articulated how I felt as we launched our married life. Although I wasn't quite like that thirty-second commercial bride, this was *my* version of a Kodak commercial.

In September we signed a mortgage on our first home—an updated 1950s rambler in Golden Valley, near my parents' house. A remodeling prior to purchase opened the galley kitchen to a living room/dining room area, and a cozy family room created a niche off the back. New tile in the kitchen, freshly painted light-colored walls, and brand-new carpeting—we loved it.

A dishwasher! What a great appliance. A garbage disposal! Amazing. Our very own washer and dryer in the basement! What a treat. The ability to paint the walls any color we wanted! Our own garage! Splendid delights in contrast to our apartment. This was that sweet spot of life when everything felt new and exciting.

We liked our new neighborhood and neighbors. To the north we had the Schnacks; to the south we had the Schnecks. Downtown Minneapolis pulsed only three miles east, the city lakes sparkled nearby, and a neighborhood park was two blocks away. A third of an acre belonged to us, and I relished the departure from our gardenless "garden" apartment. Dirk and I landscaped, planted flowers, decorated, and happily settled in. We were bona fide grown-ups.

Although only one mile existed between our new home and my childhood home at the corner of Westwood Drive and Westwood Lane, I had traveled a long way. Six years earlier, I'd slipped into reverse and longed for Seattle. My parents' home hadn't been the expected place to land, and my body's home had crumbled. But now, at the ripe old age of twenty-nine, I wasn't looking backward anymore. The home of my body still sheltered my new kidney, imperfectly, as recurrent FSGS remained inside me causing damage—but it hadn't destroyed it. And my new home with Dirk represented forward motion.

How I wanted to continue in that direction.

49

Third-Party Terrorist

BESIDES MARITAL BLISS, A FEW CHALLENGES AROSE WHEN Dirk and I fused into a shared life. Our early marriage required some adjustments, and in our first year, we started our curriculum of compromise.

For starters, there was the doormat dilemma. I purchased a "Welcome" coir doormat and placed it outside our front door. Dirk fired questions at my purchase: "When did you buy that?" Followed by, "Do we need that?" Followed by, "How much did that cost?"

What is this, an interrogation? Feeling feisty, I answered, "Yesterday." Followed by, "Yes." Followed by, "Not much." What cruised through my mind was: *Back off, bud, I'm a working woman who was capable of buying a doormat before we got married. I'll be damned if I can't buy one now.*

I imagine what was going through Dirk's mind (a guy who loves being in charge) was something like, *Oh shit, how will I manage finances when she goes off willy-nilly to buy a random doormat?*

Next up, the shower curtain incident. You heard that right; we fought over a shower curtain. Dirk had bought a shower curtain pre-marriage. And he liked it. And I didn't. I confidently rejected the shower curtain for a better one.

At first, it was like a tug-of-war. Who would decide on the myriad of things that affected us both? Feeling victorious after years of battling for independence, I didn't plan on marriage tamping that down. Dirk had been single and on his own for many years. So he didn't want to lose his independence either.

One of the better side effects of illness, my hard-won appreciate-life philosophy through gratitude, lucky lists, and positive thinking, also tripped us up. I was so indoctrinated into appreciation for the big things that I wrote off the small stuff. But Dirk cared about the small stuff and didn't appreciate my dismissal because "Hey, isn't it great to be alive!"

Eventually, we dissected what was at the heart of some of our squabbles. I heard him. If something small rubbed him wrong, like wanting me to close the cap more tightly on the toothpaste, how easy for me to accommodate that to make him happy. And he heard me too. *Don't try to control me. And by the way, I make better design decisions for our home's interior (because it's my job), and I'll be mindful of our budget.* That prompted the comment that psychology was his job, so maybe he'd make better judgments on whether I was losing it.

We established our routines. Dirk was the early riser. Not my style. Eventually, I would pull myself out of bed and shuffle into our galley kitchen. A full pot of dark-roast coffee, the way we both like it, hummed on the counter. I poured a mighty mugful and joined him at the little white table by the window that faced our backyard. He talked about the news of the day while I waited for my caffeine to kick in.

He enjoyed building his outpatient eating disorder practice and bounced ideas off me for interiors and brochure copy. I suggested he name the program after his sister, Emily, who'd developed her eating disorder when few treatment resources were available. The Emily Program was born. After Dirk took off to help people struggling with anorexia and bulimia, I showered, put on an outfit suitable for custom home clients, and headed to my office.

At each workday's end, we'd rejoin each other to catch up on the day and eat dinner. Some nights, although I'm not proud of this, we picked up Subway sandwiches and ate partial footlongs while we watched television in our family room nook. Some nights I ambitiously drowned pasta in a spicy homemade Bolognese sauce and tossed a green salad.

One evening (I served a fabulous chicken fricassee recipe, if I do say so myself), we sat together by the window, eating, talking, and listening. I felt a pang as I remembered the meal with my parents after FSGS recurred. How their life had struck me as the sum of everything wonderful and impossible to achieve. I smiled as Dirk told me some details about his day.

"What?" he asked. My smile was too generous for his topic, so he knew I was thinking about something else.

"Nothing," I said. "Just thinking . . . what a wonderful world."

"Cheers to that," he agreed, and we clinked our glasses.

Rachael shared the joyful news that she was pregnant, and many of my friends also began planning families. I imagined having babies too. A jolt traveled through me when I remembered the doctors had considered giving me that medication that could have made me sterile. If indeed I could get pregnant, that memory would be just an echo—a near miss without devastating contact. The thought made me shiver, like I'd dodged a bullet.

Even so, I never pursued medical information on getting pregnant; I'd steamrolled into our marriage, assuming I'd be healthy and have a child. FSGS wasn't hereditary, so I forged ahead, figuring everything would magically align with my dreams of a normal, meaningful life.

Dirk, however, seemed more ambivalent, and we didn't have

a well-crafted family plan before we got married. We'd talked about kids sometimes in an imaginary and aspirational way, but never in a when-and-how-many way. One evening, after I checked in on how Rae was feeling, I asked Dirk, "Do you wonder what our kids will look like?"

Side by side in our den, we sunk comfortably into the soft cushions. "Jen, we don't have to have kids," he said, pivoting his position to face me. "A lot of couples don't have children, and they're happy. I'm okay if that's the way it goes for us." He widened his eyes and measured mine.

"Don't you want to have kids?" I asked. My voice and body tightened as I sat up straight. *Am I going to have to talk him into this? Wasn't this the implied plan all along?*

"I can go either way. I'm just saying if it isn't a good idea, we can accept that." He looked straight at me and held my gaze. His eyes softened with compassion.

"No, I can't accept that," I said, and shook my head. "There's no other way. I need to be a mom." Then I expanded with determination because I realized the power of my drive to nurture a child. I wanted to experience the other side of the close bond that I shared with my mom, and I couldn't picture my future without a child to love.

"Okay," Dirk replied. "And if it doesn't work, we'll be fine. Just the two of us." He put his hand on mine. I wondered if he believed that. Or did he fear complications? We had fine-tuned our system of compromise at this point by yielding to whoever felt the strongest about an issue, and clearly, I housed strong feelings about having children.

"It will all work out," I said. I'd shoved aside the reality that I had a transplanted kidney that wouldn't last forever, and my health would remain a chronic issue. But I'd voiced my intentions. To Dirk. To the universe. I would be a mom someday.

He nodded, but I wasn't convinced he believed my statement. Did he think I wouldn't be able to have a baby? And was he softening me for that possibility?

One thing we knew, a third party always lurked nearby: destructive autoimmunity. Not in ways we dealt with every day—more like a terrorist who lived in the attic. That terrorist kept to himself for many years, but we understood he hovered and could, at any time, surface with a destructive blast.

50

Accumulation

A YEAR PASSED. WHILE OUR MARRIAGE GREW STRONGER, my kidney function grew weaker. My weight dropped and tipped me into the too-thin range. Despite exhaustion, I kept up with my job. My clients distracted me, helpfully so, from the inevitable kidney fade that would lead me back to a dialysis machine.

This time, it was a slow slide, as opposed to a rapid decline. But everything felt like an effort, from getting dressed and out the door, to pushing up from a chair in the conference room to leave a meeting. Sluggish. Low energy. No appetite. Mental fog. Always chilly, but medications kept the swelling under control.

My "acting" skills came in handy at work. Frequently, I dragged myself to a client meeting and then tapped into an inexplicable hidden reserve to keep up my professionalism. As if I heard "showtime," I could suddenly perform on stage.

Right after our first anniversary, Dirk and I traveled to his Pennsylvania hometown to celebrate his mom's sixty-fifth birthday. The sun shone as we enjoyed birthday cake, ice cream, and Miller family dynamics on my brother-in-law's farm. I took in the green rolling hills and allowed my anemic body to find peace in the quiet rural setting.

I remembered when Dirk and I had started dating, before I'd even met his parents, his mom (a nurse) cautioned him about traipsing into my dangerous minefield. Knowing her initial concerns had made me extra self-conscious during her first visit to Minneapolis.

As our introductory dinner, Dirk's dad, Merv, a quiet spectacled man, wore an even expression to show his gentle disposition. Dirk's mom, Arlene, an engaging conversationalist, peppered our meal with lively discussions about interesting books she'd read, curious questions about my interests, my friends, and my sense of style. She complimented me lavishly on my clothing and hair. She inquired about my family and job. Grays peppered her wavy brown bob, the sun she loved made its mark on her skin, and Talbots inspired her outfit. She was a lovely woman.

Curiously, she repeated this statement three times: "You are not a mother, so you don't know this. But when your child hurts, you hurt too."

I wondered why she had kept saying this to me. Was her message, *You hurt my kid, you hurt me?* Had she regarded me as a ticking bomb that could hurt her son? That thought stirred up the sadness I'd tried to escape.

But as for her concern about Dirk hooking up with my damaged self, truthfully, could I blame her? Hadn't I shared the same concerns? After she'd expressed her worries to Dirk, eventually she said to him, "I know my son. You'll marry her anyway."

Later, after Dirk announced our engagement to his family, his mom responded, "Well, if that is your decision, then we will love her too."

I'd let that shaken snow globe of guilt and fear settle back into a resting state. And now, as Dirk and I tucked one year of marriage under our belt, we celebrated Arlene's milestone birthday in the sunshine on that farm. She focused on me with all the love she'd promised to deliver and asked about my health. "You're very thin," she said with visible worry. "How are you?"

Arlene's nurse vocabulary made it easy to discuss details about my kidney health. She told me she admired my positivity, squeezed my arm with affection, and spilled genuine love. But I hesitated to accept it because her love felt framed in pity. I rejected pity, equating it to a neon sign flashing the words "You're pathetic."

Dirk and I would get through this, and we'd be okay. I wanted her and everyone to realize we would not get blown up stepping through medical minefields. I defended Dirk's decision to choose me, in emotional self-defense, so I didn't have to consider if she'd been right about me from the start.

The week after we returned from Pennsylvania in late June 1995, I accumulated water weight rapidly. The kidney had run its course, and I called Dr. Brown. "It's time—let's put you back on the transplant list, start treatments three times a week, and get you feeling better." Dr. Brown rang the bell, and my second round of dialysis commenced.

Oh no, not again. What would our lives be like now? A wintry dread filled my gut as I returned to a place I didn't want to go.

———

PART FOUR

ACCEPTING

"Fall down seven times, stand up eight."

—Japanese proverb

51.

Dogs + Dialysis

AS I SAT WITH DR. BROWN IN HIS OFFICE, HE WRAPPED up our appointment with this: "I have some news. I'm going to retire." His announcement caught me off guard. I'd never considered such a thing. Could he actually do that?

"My wife and I are moving to Santa Fe," he explained. "It seems like the right time. I know you'll be in excellent hands with one of our other nephrologists."

"Well, it's been great working with you," I said, and heard how cheesy it sounded, like we'd been insurance colleagues with an impersonal connection. The truth was, he'd led me through a searing fire with his expert care and tended those high flames until they became low-burning embers. We'd navigated through intense stuff together. He seemed a tad melancholy, but his decision to retire from his practice was a big one.

Although he had lots of other patients, I had only one Dr. Brown. How would I do this without his eyes peering at me through those oval metal-rimmed glasses—carefully evaluating my medications and protocols? What would kidney management look like without his tweed jackets, bow ties, and professorial manner, so focused on my case?

Dr. Brown's retirement announcement amplified the loneliness of my illness. I wanted to retire from kidney problems as easily as he planned to retire from nephrology. I'd love to change my scenery, but wherever I went, FSGS tagged along.

What about Dirk? Might he retire from my illness? We were married, sure, but marriages end all the time. If he left, my disease would be out of his life. And Mom? As much as she'd sealed our souls and never left me to suffer alone, what if something happened to her? And Dad? At day's end, I *was* alone, no matter how you sliced it. The tormentor of autoimmunity affected us all, and simultaneously it remained all mine. This realization permeated like a botched tattoo inked into my thoughts.

Even in kindergarten, I had considered my singular place amongst others in the world. One night, way back then, tucked under my blanket, I tried to comprehend that I'd only be me. Of all the people in the world, I would always stay confined within myself. I underwent a five-year-old's existential crisis as I pondered my individual boundaries. It's a big thought for a kid who should have been thinking about riding a bike or running through the sprinklers. If I could go back in time, I would tell myself to chillax.

For the fun of it, I recreated altered versions of myself. There was the Carmelita name stage, because really, Carmelita Cramer, how fun is that to say? That didn't stick. I changed the spelling of Jenny to Jennie for a while. A temporary diversion. I "changed" my middle name from Mary to Marie. My mom rolled with it as I came home with school projects labeled with an assortment of different spellings. Now my trippy little girl ideas to expand beyond myself magnified in my mind by a thousand. How remarkable would it feel to step outside the constraints of my skin?

When Dr. Brown left, Dr. Somermeyer took over. He was taller, younger, equally smart, and ready to manage my care. His intensity gave me confidence. My dialysis location changed from Abbott to Methodist Hospital, and my previous two-hour treatment extended to the same three and a half hours as in Seattle—

again, because studies showed longer dialysis is easier on the body.

Two favorable differences made the start of dialysis round two better than round one: 1) my fistula was in place, so I didn't require a rogue country-singing surgeon to place it, and 2) I hadn't been taking prednisone, so all those earlier side effects were nonexistent. I asked Dr. Somermeyer if the length of my kidney run seemed a disappointment, and he underscored the value of all I'd achieved with the first kidney:

It was a successful five-year-and-three-month dialysis vacation.

1,915 days.

47,960 hours.

2,777,600 minutes.

I pondered his perspective. My donor had provided years, months, days, hours, minutes that allowed me to build a career, earn a master's degree, unite in marriage, and share a home. For this, I danced with gratitude.

Happy things, yes, yes, yes. But an element of grief and despair flared. A sense of loss. Just as my marriage was getting underway, I needed another transplant. Every cell in my body cried out, *No, no, no. Please, give me a break!* I wept privately in the shower because I wanted to hide all the thoughts that weren't positive. This had become my forte. Even though I knew better, I didn't give all my emotions equal weight. I fought to repel the fear, but it seeped in. I didn't want to do this all over again. It scared me. Was this body of mine, this make and model, equipped to withstand another onslaught?

I was about to find out.

I typically arrived at the hospital after work, stopped at the first-floor coffee shop, and bought a low-fat lemon muffin. Up on the third floor, I entered the unit and sat in a reclining dialysis chair for the long haul. I passed the time by catching *Entertainment Tonight*, prime time to follow, and savored that lemon muffin. Nibble by nibble. A coping technique: pair a reward with something unpleasant. In this case, dialysis was a drag, but that muffin . . . now *that* was delicious.

Here's the deal with chronic illness—you learn to better absorb its ups and downs. You hear women talking about the difference between a first and second pregnancy, and how the experience morphs from big deal to been-there-doing-it-again. Baby-making is still worthy of complaints, but you've done the drill. That's how dialysis round two felt, sort of. But unlike pregnancy, dialysis kept me alive, and there wasn't a tangible nine-month limit to the experience. I might wait six months or three years for another kidney; I had no way to know.

FSGS recurrence is like a well-worn knife. It still cuts, but not as deep. Still . . . ouch. My skin became thicker, but maintaining positivity became a continuous practice. Some days came easier than others.

My health was retreating again. But I remembered Dr. Brown's words to Dirk after we got married. And I wanted to prove them true. I owed it to Dirk. A bother, not a burden.

Dirk and I talked about getting a dog and decided on a wheaten terrier (like Mickey, my parents' dialysis-inspired dog). We met a breeder named Earl, picked out a frisky puppy, and called her Zoe. She was eight weeks old when we brought her home in a little plastic crate.

Zoe whined at night, peed, pooped, and chewed. Good thing she was adorable. A four-legged distraction I could love. When I felt tired after a day of working with demanding clients and dialysis machines, Zoe didn't care—she still wanted to lick my face and run around in circles. Now two wheaten terrier puppies had entered my life when I started each round of dialysis, first Mickey and now Zoe. Coping with dogs became an emerging pattern, and puppy wonders eased medical bummers.

But my Zoe, positivity practice, and survival instincts couldn't erase the challenges I faced. Back to the fluid and food restrictions—and to the realization that I was alive because some super-smart person had invented this artificial kidney machine.

If I'd been alive in the 1950s, my predicament would have been a death sentence. In the early sixties, the first outpatient dialysis clinic opened in Seattle with only six machines. This posed a significant moral dilemma for doctors. They rationed the life-saving procedure, and many people died. A 1965 documentary by NBC News, *Who Shall Live*, detailed the selection process for these first dialysis patients "lucky" enough to live in Seattle.

First, a committee of Seattle doctors tested the potential patients' medical fitness to survive the rigors of the dialysis process. In those days, the treatment lasted an agonizing twelve to sixteen hours. In contrast, today's more typical three-to-four-hour treatments seem like a piece of cake.

The next hurdle involved a psychological evaluation. Did the patient have the courage to undergo the process? Did the patient have the stamina to live this way and endure multiple hours in a hospital bed?

The third step required a meeting with a financial committee. How would the applicant pay for the procedure? The cost was $10,000 a year and patients paid three years of fees upfront. To put that in perspective, $10,000 in 1962, adjusted for inflation, is equal to approximately $96,000 in 2023, and the three-year upfront payment would equal about $288,000.

If the medical, psychological, and financial committees approved the patient, a volunteer jury of peers weighed in on the overarching record of this person in the community. Was this applicant worth saving? It is staggering to imagine what these patients faced.

No committees evaluated if my life was worth saving. And in 1972, under President Nixon's administration, ten years after those Seattle selection panels, Congress approved Medicare coverage for dialysis and kidney transplants, regardless of age. When this program folded into the Social Security Act, the life and death panels that determined treatment eligibility disappeared.

When my kidneys reached the end stage, Medicare kicked in. And again, I must acknowledge—I know how lucky I am. Without the resources available to me, my access to supplemental insurance and Medicare, this journey would have been infinitely more difficult. Among all these things, my family didn't face financial devastation.

When I considered how far dialysis had come, it helped me redirect my thoughts in a more positive direction. At least I had access to solutions. And although dialysis is a tough way to live, it was the *only* way to live absent a transplant. Dialysis for me equaled life. And life was everything.

52

Call #2

FIVE MONTHS LATER, ON A BRISK NOVEMBER MORNING in 1995, I hustled down the hall to pick up the ringing phone. On the line, a doctor from the university said, "Hi, Jennifer. We have an excellent kidney for you. It's close to a perfect match. Can you come in and get it?" He sounded so matter-of-fact. Did he think I might have something better to do?

"Of course!" I said as my knees buckled.

Is this really happening? I tipped my head back, raised my palms to the ceiling, and inhaled a generous breath. For three seconds, I steadied myself. Then I buzzed into action.

I flung open the front door and artic Minnesota air slapped my face. I screamed to Dirk as he shoveled snow in the driveway. Surrounded by flying white powder, he'd wintered up with Sorel boots, a puffy jacket, and heavy-duty leather gloves.

"Dirk! They have a good kidney for me!"

The shovel flew. He rushed in, shed the winter wear, and shifted straightaway into his hyper-focused gear. I could see it in his rapid movements and tightened lips. We quickly shoved a bag with hospital essentials and arranged care for Zoe. Then we called my parents, interrupting their vacation in the Cayman Islands, to tell them the news.

"You ready?" Dirk asked. His face broadcast mixed signals of determination with a helpless fear that edged his eyes.

"I'm ready. Let's go get a kidney." Butterflies fluttered in my stomach as my heartbeat rose in my throat.

"Grab my arm. I don't want you to slip on the ice," Dirk said as we walked out the front door. I crooked my arm into the safety of his bent elbow, and together we walked to the car. I knew what was in store. Surgery. Wake up. Hope my new kidney would work right away. Pain. Hope it would continue to work. Heal. But this time it felt different because Dirk was there.

"If you want to get there fast," he said, "you're with the right guy." I typically cringed at his lead-foot speeds, but on this occasion, I wasn't going to complain. I knew his tight grip and focus on the snowy road would help him shut out the distracting voices of worry.

Meanwhile, my mom and dad tried to get on a flight home as soon as possible.

Within an hour, nurses prepped me in the pre-surgery area. The sterile environment and fluorescent assault amplified my agitation. Dirk held my hand. The anesthesiologist approached with a syringe; I felt Dirk's grip squeeze firmly as the sedation hit my vein. And . . . out. I can imagine what Dirk did during the four-hour operation to fend off a bombardment of anxiety. Pacing. Filling Styrofoam cups with lousy coffee. Short, repetitive phone conversations to repeat that he'd heard nothing yet.

I woke up to Dirk's amplified voice. "The kidney worked on the table. You've been peeing like a racehorse!" I attempted a smile, but the medicated haze and midsection pain dulled my reaction. I fell back into a cloudy slumber. Later, I awoke in my room and heard buzzing machines, the rumble of rolling scales through the halls, and the chatter of nurses at the station outside my door. My husband stood at the ready with a pitcher of ice chips and a wide-toothed grin, showcasing his relief.

"Let me help you," he volunteered when the time came for my first post-surgery shower. He steadied me as I stood, just as he'd done earlier on that icy sidewalk.

"Here goes," I said as he untied the back of my flimsy hospital gown. It fell onto the bathroom floor to reveal the fresh boomerang-shaped incision opposite my first faded transplant scar. Together, Dirk and I wrestled the clinging polyester curtain and lifted the handheld shower spray. The liters of IV fluid they'd pumped into me to profuse the new kidney had distended my abdomen. My body's midsection felt like a waterbed. I turned to show him my fresh wound. "Check it out, dude."

His eyes flooded with a look I'll never forget. Like a romanticized diamond commercial, his gaze suggested I was the most beautiful woman in the world. How he pulled that look off, I'll never know. His promise was tested . . . for better or worse. A+.

We all knew recurrence could show up again (#incurable), but unlike my first transplant, I did not spill a large quantity of protein immediately after my surgery. Let me repeat that. I did *not* spill a ton of protein. For now. And *now* was what I had. A deep tension cracked opened within me, and relief filled that space. Maybe, just maybe, things would perfectly align this time. A girl could hope.

A new transplant vacation was underway; I spent five days and four nights in the hospital. I never received information about the donor. Perhaps the family wanted privacy. But I released my most potent prayer to ease the sadness of their horrific loss. And I sent gratitude for their life-changing generosity.

Later, I would become a volunteer ambassador for Donate Life, a nonprofit organization dedicated to increasing donation and saving lives through transplants. I would speak to groups about the overwhelming goodness of organ donors and explain that one person can save and heal up to seventy-five lives. And I would learn donor families often share that their loved one's donation comforts them through their grief journey. It's an indescribable privilege to hold kidneys in my body from people who checked a box because they wanted to pay forward the gift of life.

When we arrived home, I walked in the front door, and Zoe ran up to greet me. I petted her while taking in the fragrant flowers that friends and family had sent to our home.

I dried the blooms and used them to decorate our Christmas tree. Roses, hydrangea, and a variety of beautiful petals tucked in between evergreen needles. It served as a visible reminder of the new kidney and all the people we loved. "You've decorated wonderful trees before," Dirk said. "But this one is my favorite."

53.

White Stick

SEVEN MONTHS LATER, A SATURDAY IN MAY, MY energy seemed to wash away in the shower. Inexplicably drained, I grabbed the remote, called Zoe over to nestle by my side, and hit the couch. I'd been dog-tired before, but this was double-strength exhaustion. I was in the critical post-transplant window (under a year) and needed to report anything that "didn't feel right." Because I was at high risk for rejection, my exhaustion ushered in a fear-edged unease.

Dirk saw a few clients in the morning, hit the golf course in the afternoon, and returned to find me in the same unproductive lounging state. We'd planned to go to a party that evening. But I couldn't do it.

"Are you okay?" Dirk asked, walking over to the couch with taut brows. "What's going on?" He sat down next to me and stared into my face for clues.

"Sorry . . . I'm so tired. Count me out, but you go," I said.

"Wow, okay," he replied, sounding uneasy. "I'll represent us and stay for a bit. You rest." After he kissed me goodbye on the forehead, I breathed a deep relief knowing that I'd stay put.

The overriding exhaustion continued. As the days trudged on, peculiar smells repulsed me. Driving down the road, the smell of asphalt nearly did me in. Then I had a field day with a jar of pickles. You can guess where this is going. Stereotypical as it sounds, the taste of those sodium-soaked cucumbers was irresistible.

Beth stopped into town to see her family and asked if I wanted to join her for dinner. As we caught up, I didn't mention that I hadn't had a period in the seven months since I'd received my transplant. Initially, I brushed it off as a post-surgery body adjustment, but the exhaustion, newfound pickle passion, and super sensitive breasts pointed to signs I couldn't ignore. On the way home, I scooped up a pregnancy test.

Beelining into our bathroom, I peed on the white stick. Wait, wait, wait. I looked. There it was—a little blue cross—positively pregnant. An audible gasp escaped my mouth. So that explained it! Something *was* going on with my body. My excitement landed somewhere between winning the lottery and a grand karmic gift to fulfill my destiny. I bolted down the hall and joined Dirk in the family room, where a baseball game had absorbed him.

"I think I'm pregnant?" I said with a rising inflection that mirrored my hesitation (and made me sound like a Valley girl). Dirk remained in his baseball-induced trance.

"Why do you think that?" he asked, looking up for a split second. His attention remained divided. I'd say 20 percent me, 80 percent boys of summer.

"I took a test. It's positive!" I was on the verge of doing a cartwheel.

"From the drugstore?"

"Yes!"

"Those over-the-counter tests aren't very accurate," he replied. *How does he know anything about pregnancy tests?* With that dismissal, he continued to watch base runners and bat swingers. I cocked my head and let out an intentionally loud, frustrated sigh.

I marched to the bedroom and called my mom. When she picked up, I quickly blurted out, "Hey, guess what? I might be pregnant."

Her reply? "Oh, come on. You're not pregnant."

Another skeptic. Why didn't anyone believe me? Yes, my body had been through a roller coaster of dialysis and surgery, and it wasn't conducive to a period. Did that warrant zero faith in my child-conceiving ability? Apparently so. Dirk and my mom didn't seem able to allow that idea into their minds.

I called Dawn next, and she said, "If the test is positive, you're pregnant." Finally, someone listened to me! With an electric charge of exhilaration, I smiled so hard my cheeks stretched. Truthfully, I understood Dirk's and Mom's initial reactions—I hadn't tried to prevent it because I assumed my body wouldn't readily accept a pregnancy. So if baby-making was possible, I'd figured it would take a long time. Although I was determined to have a child one day, it was unbelievable *that* day was starting on *this* day!

Transplant doctors discourage pregnancy in the first year after surgery because the high medication doses can harm a developing baby. Plus, the additional stress on the body can present a greater risk to a new kidney. I was five months short of a year when my ob-gyn confirmed what I already knew. It was official. Preggers.

I quickly made an appointment with Dr. Somermeyer to confess my tomfoolery. When I told him, he congratulated me and offered a half smile. (He wasn't a bounteous smiler.) "I was afraid you'd be mad at me," I said.

"Of course not. *I'm* going to manage your medications, and *you're* going to have a baby." Hearing those words out loud, "You're going to have a baby," lifted me right up. I practically bounced out of his clinic.

At my office, I readily beamed the news to my coworkers. One day, I plopped down in the chair on the opposite side of my dad's sturdy desk, moved a pile of files to the side, and rambled joyfully about my baby excitement. Out of sync with my pumped-up energy, Dad wore a serious expression. "I don't think you should tell many people yet," he said quietly.

"Why?" I asked. But I knew why. He immediately traveled forward in his mind and envisioned me having to tell people I wasn't pregnant anymore. It was such a different response than I wanted. Was this his Dale Carnegie think-the-worst technique playing out with my baby? I sat forward, rigid in my seat.

"It'll be fine, Dad. I know it." It unsteadied me that he would suggest something so negative. *Where did Mr. Positive go?*

That evening at home, I told Dirk what my dad had said. I assumed Dirk, at least, would fully share my enthusiasm. *We* were going to have a baby!

"I get what your dad's saying. I don't want to be excited yet either," Dirk said, leaning back in his chair.

"How can you *not* be excited?" I practically shouted.

"If something goes wrong . . ." He paused. "I don't want to get excited until I know it's going to be okay." Our energies didn't match. He sunk down low, and I rose to cloud nine.

"But Dirk, don't you get it? *This is* the moment to be excited. This is it!" I explained. "If I'm not pregnant sometime in the future, if anything terrible happens, we'll lose the chance to feel this way—we must be excited *now*. Because *now*, at this very moment—regardless of what happens down the road—I AM PREGNANT!" His reluctance seemed equivalent to ignoring a gorgeous day because you never know if it may rain.

I recalled Tom's death as a reminder that you never know what's in store—so embrace what you have now. If this pregnancy amounted to thirty minutes of wonderful, I would take it.

Even if others didn't feel the same, I couldn't contain my joy. *I did it, I did it—we did it!* If pregnancy truly creates a glow, I sparkled like a firefly in a dark night sky. *Look at me, on track to have full membership in the ordinary life club!* What was more "normal" than being married with a job, a dog, and a baby on board?

I held tight to the notion that just like life, pregnancy was black-and-white. My kidney transplant did not make me less pregnant. Being 100 percent pregnant, I decided to appreciate every pregnant day I had.

The secret of health for both the body and the mind is not to mourn the past or worry about the future, but to live in the present moment wisely and earnestly.

—Buddha

54

Little Life

AT MY FIRST PRENATAL VISIT, I MET MY REMARKABLE ob-gyn, Dr. Virginia Lupo, a specialist in high-risk pregnancies. Dr. Lupo's outgoing personality put me at ease, and her successful experience with difficult deliveries felt both reassuring and encouraging.

"My primary concern is high blood pressure. It can happen during pregnancy and would be hard on your kidney," she said. "We'll keep a close eye on that." I'd become accustomed to taking my blood pressure at home, so that'd be easy to monitor.

"I'm also wondering where that baby will grow with all those extra parts in there," she continued. (I had two transplanted kidneys positioned in the front, one of which worked, and my two original kidneys in the back.) "But the body is accommodating, so I'm confident those organs will shift around to make room for your little cupcake."

Twelve weeks had already passed before I discovered my pregnant status, so my first trimester sailed by before I realized it had begun. I read about the miracle of pregnancy and the week-by-week process of development. I had grand confidence that eyes and limbs would form, limb buds would grow into hands and feet, and the heart, lungs, brain, mouth, eyes, and spinal cord would develop correctly.

Like healing, I knew my body would take over and form a perfect baby. I used my creative visualization techniques and let the wonder take place inside of me. What's more life-affirming than my life (with significant help from Dirk) creating life? Steve was right about the body's ability to handle a lot. *Move aside, Eric Clapton, I'm pregnant!* And the gift of life I'd received from my donor was also the gift that enabled me to create a new life.

My mom came with me for my next visit. I heard my baby's heartbeat through a microphone. *Whoosh. Whoosh. Whoosh.* The sound of life beat inside me. And I saw it/him/her/baby—black, gray, and white. Surreal compositions outlined a baby head, baby arms, and baby legs. It was real and unreal at once, and I expanded with an immense sense of accomplishment.

My mom smiled too. "What a wonder," she said.

I remembered my verbal outburst the evening Dirk had proposed. We could have a dog! We could have a house! We could have a kid! Check one. Check two. Now . . . check three on the way. At thirty-one, I somehow lived amidst my visualizations. I couldn't wait to be a mom.

When Dirk and I attended our four-and-a-half-month ultrasound, I felt it deep in the fibers of my being—my growing baby would appear perfectly healthy. I was right. Dr. Lupo saw a heart beating with four chambers, kidneys, hands, feet, a smiling face, and a little moving mouth. She also identified girl parts.

"Are you sure?" I asked with hesitation. (A friend's doctor stated the sex of her baby and claimed a fifty-fifty chance of being right. I was hoping for more accuracy.)

"I can see that little hamburger bun perfectly," Dr. Lupo said buoyantly. "You will have a girl, without a doubt." Hmm . . . an interesting affinity she had for baked goods. Our little cupcake now looked like a hamburger bun.

As I looked at Dirk, his eyes misted, and his mouth quivered. "I was hoping for a girl," he said. Tears welled up in my eyes too.

I thought of my mom and hoped that I could provide my daughter the same incredible closeness. I had big motherhood shoes to fill.

The name game soon began. Dirk ruled out many of my ideas because he'd either dated a girl with that name or treated her for a mental illness. He wanted to name our daughter Zoe, which seemed silly because our dog was Zoe. He proposed we change our dog's name to Jo-Jo, but I rejected that idea. It seemed too complicated to explain to the Schnecks and Schnacks. ("Don't call Zoe 'Zoe' because our daughter is Zoe, so now Zoe is Jo-Jo.")

We borrowed Dr. Lupo's "cupcake" nickname, because I loved hearing her exclaim, "The little cupcake is doing great!" Finally, we chose the name Liza—a combination of Mom's name, Elizabeth, and a relative of Dirk's named Eliza. Her name would be new and old, honor family bonds, and offer a fresh start. My little person, Liza Miller, was on her way to join our family. I felt ready and capable of nurturing this new life forever.

55

A Kink

AT TWENTY WEEKS, MY BABY BUMP POPPED, AND my budding basketball felt awkward in my body. Dressing for a neighborhood party one evening, I spent an inordinate amount of time trying to find something cute to wear. I grappled with my options and finally settled on a black linen shirt.

Okay, this will do. Mission accomplished. I emerged from the bedroom, relieved. "I'm ready to go," I announced.

Dirk said lovingly, "Wow . . . I can see our baby! You're showing!" I did not register the loving part; instead, I burst into tears. Didn't he know how hard it was to assemble an outfit that made me look less pregnant? I surged with hormones, and my emotions popped right along with my bump. He offered an instant hug and smirked at my unpredictable mix of pregnancy elation and emotionality. *How would he feel if his hormonal body was sprouting a person?*

Our little cupcake kept growing, and I adjusted to my expanding belly. As I drove around in my car, I belted out songs and basked in the happiness of being pregnant. I also played "The Ash Grove" on the piano. (My parents had no use for their piano anymore, so we had placed it in our living room by the fireplace.) This song from my childhood piano lessons and wedding ceremony became the melodic backdrop to my pregnancy.

But at twenty-eight weeks, I fought recurrent urinary tract infections. Dr. Lupo gave me safe antibiotics for use with Liza, but the pesky infections continued. Dr. Somermeyer investigated further. He hospitalized me and ran tests. An ultrasound revealed the baby was pushing on my ureter, the tube that connects the kidney and bladder. The ureter is essentially a hose; my hose had a kink, and fluid was backing up into my kidney. Dr. Somermeyer discharged me with continued antibiotics and instructed me to take it easy for the rest of the pregnancy.

Before I left, a nurse informed me about the potential complications of premature birth. The list was unfathomable. When she spoke of cerebral palsy, intellectual disability, respiratory distress, and bleeding into the brain, tremendous fear seized me from head to toe. But no. *No.* That would not be the case here. I rejected that possibility.

Slightly over thirty weeks, my body felt different. I didn't know what'd changed, exactly. No spotting. No cramping. Nothing physical. But an intuitive unease swept through me. I'd learned to listen to my body and act quickly when something felt off. So I rushed in to see Dr. Lupo.

"You have a premature rupture in the membrane sac that is holding your baby," she said. "You've lost amniotic fluid and have a slow leak."

My body clenched with a sudden chill. "Oh my God, what does that mean?" I asked.

"It means you need to be on bed rest immediately. I'm concerned about infection risk and premature delivery." Fear invaded my thoughts and muscles, and as if hit with an unexpected punch, I bent over to catch my breath.

Premature deliveries were common in transplant patient

pregnancies. I had read that. But the difference between reading this and being told to go lie down immediately was night and day. I had to protect my baby, and I wanted Liza to stay inside and develop until she was ready to be born.

"Our next step is to schedule an amniocentesis to determine if your daughter's lungs are developed," Dr. Lupo said. I wanted to shout, *My daughter's name is Liza,* to emphasize she was a real girl with an actual name and she had to be okay. The doctor explained that as soon as Liza's lungs were ready to breathe without assistance, the best thing for both of us would be an induction.

The results came back. Liza's lungs had not developed enough yet. If born with lungs in this condition, she'd require a ventilator and face potential complications for survival. I remembered the panic that had overcome me when my lungs filled with fluid years earlier. *Oh, God, no.* Her sweet, tiny lungs needed strength. The unthinkable horror of her gasping for air petrified me.

While it was not safe for her yet in the outside world, the slow leak of amniotic fluid posed a risk to her inside world. Dr. Lupo's job was to balance both threats, and she recommended I return in a week to reevaluate with a repeat amniocentesis.

Dirk set me up on the couch in the television niche. I had blankets, tissues, a remote control, a pitcher of water, snacks, books, magazines, and a journal. Hot tears poured down my cheeks while on bed rest. Two episodes of kidney failure and two kidney transplants had done nothing to prepare me for the panic that my baby might not be okay.

Dread pumped through my body like a secondary blood system, an all-encompassing liquid fear that polluted my cells. I'd developed highly refined skills in dealing with health issues confined within *my* body. *My* life. This was beyond me.

My faithful companion, Zoe, positioned her warm body next to me, and I petted her repeatedly to soften my stress. Mom visited during the long days. At night, Dirk joined me on the couch. My partner in fear and anxiety, Dirk served dinner on trays and massaged my feet.

"Do you feel anything? Has she been moving?" he said, putting his hand on my belly. "She'll be born soon. I can't believe it."

"Not too soon, I hope." The longer my baby developed inside me, the better. But Dirk seemed misguidedly gung-ho, as if the sooner she was born, the sooner we'd be parents. While he didn't get how serious prematurity problems could be, I felt a crushing responsibility. I had to make sure she was all right.

Seven days passed. Dr. Lupo didn't know how much longer I could keep Liza inside with the loss of amniotic fluid. She scheduled the second amniocentesis for the afternoon to determine the condition of her lungs.

Imagining my baby in jeopardy was incomprehensible. If something happened to her, I wouldn't be able to endure it. My pregnancy occurred ahead of the recommended guidelines. Was this part of an irresponsible push forward to have a normal life? Had I undertaken one risk too many?

The upcoming test results were critical.

Dirk and I drove to the Hennepin County Medical Center. After the test, we returned home immediately, and I resumed bed rest. Zoe nestled in again by my side, and Dirk and I waited for the call to learn if Liza's lungs permitted a next day delivery.

Waiting was torture. Spirals of anxiety twisted inside me like a taut elastic band.

A ring. Dirk answered the phone. I stared at his face as Dr. Lupo spoke to him. He nodded, and his lips curled. Then he looked at me and held his thumb up in the air. "Her lung development has increased significantly since last week, and the cupcake is ready to be born without ventilation!" he said, repeating Dr. Lupo's words out loud.

"Oh," I gasped, and put my hand over my mouth.

"We're going to have our baby tomorrow, Jen. It's going to be okay!" he exclaimed through happy tears. We hugged each other tightly with elation and frenzy.

Liza would join us within twenty-four hours, although she would go straight to the neonatal intensive care unit (NICU). I inhaled a big breath, and my fears vaporized. Now I felt it deep within my gut. Our baby girl would be all right.

It never occurred to me *I* might not be all right.

56

A Rush

MY NESTING INSTINCTS TOOK OVER WHOLEHEARTEDLY, and I couldn't stay confined on the couch anymore. I figured who needs bed rest when the next day would be our daughter's predetermined birthday? I tidied in a frenzied attempt to have everything in place. Perfection was shouting at me, *Get ready! You must be completely prepared!*

Liza's room already contained a maple crib, sweet bedding, a changing table, the Diaper Genie, and a small love seat.

"Dirk, we never got her room painted," I said with overblown remorse. The walls weren't right. (As if our baby would notice the color of the room.) Suddenly, it seemed as critical as her lung development. And even though I knew she wouldn't come home right away, my nesting instincts went wild.

I called my mom and dad right after we received the predetermined birthday news. Mom planned to arrive at the hospital later in the day to relieve Dirk. I called back again, and my dad answered.

"I'm really upset about Liza's room," I told him, dumping my words with urgency.

"What about it?" he asked.

"It's not ready; we never painted it. The room is not ready!"

"Would you feel better if Steve and I picked up some paint and came over?" Dad asked, his patience and generosity coming to the rescue.

Steve was in town for the Christmas holiday. Still a single New Yorker, he had shelved his screenwriting aspirations to accept a job developing software applications for his alma mater.

"Yes! Thank you so much, Dad. Sorry if this is crazy, but I'm panicked, and I'd be so grateful!"

"Don't worry, Jenny. What color?"

The color that had imparted good health to my acupuncturist's room, the color that had soothed me in my apartment with Beth and housed me after my first transplant—I knew just the color that would keep my baby safe.

"Super soft pink," I said. So Dad and Steve came over with paint cans, rollers, brushes, and a tarp. And within a short time, the walls became pinkified. Who else but family can you show your most emotional craziness to, and they try to make it okay?

Dirk and I got to bed early. Dr. Lupo's team expected us at 6:30 a.m. to start the induction. In the middle of the night, I woke up to use the bathroom. Heavy-duty cramps made me sit on the edge of the tub to catch my breath. The pains continued off and on through the night. I'd never had internal pain before that elicited a deep moan, an attachment of sound to feeling.

In the morning, Dirk gathered our things, and we left for the hospital. We packed a CD player and a stack of my favorite music. We expected a long day and picked a scenic mental image to help me through the contractions. Since Dirk and I loved our honeymoon, we decided I'd picture the South of France to escape from labor pains. Specifically, we chose the view in Saint-Jean-Cap-Ferrat, where sapphire-blue water lapped against rocky outcroppings, the sun beamed, and a cloudless sky opened above us.

Far from France, however, we faced a frigid Minnesota morning, three days before Christmas 1996, while a band of heavy snow fell. Arm in arm, we walked to the car. I hunched over and said, "These cramps are painful." I groaned as I fully reclined in the back seat. Dirk focused on the road as he raced through the empty snowy streets, ambulance-driver style, to get to Hennepin County Medical Center.

When we arrived at the maternity floor, I calmed down, knowing I'd soon be in Dr. Lupo's expert hands. Several nurses rushed into my room and made me comfortable. I tucked into the bed and waited for the show to begin. Here I was—in another hospital room. But my kidney had nothing to do with it. This time, I checked in to give birth to a promising new human.

Straightaway, a nurse informed me that my "cramps" signaled real-deal contractions. Dirk held my hand, and I clenched my jaw through the pain. When the contraction ended, the pain subsided. And Dirk and I filled the in-between space with animated conversations about our life ahead as parents. Then another contraction seized me, and we progressed through the pain again, knowing it was temporary and I could handle it. It occurred to me these contractions resembled how we navigate the troublesome times in our lives. We endure them. They pass. We carry on.

Soon, the contractions fired closer together. With a concerned look, my nurse asked, "Jennifer, do you feel you want to push?"

"Sort of," I said, "but . . . I don't know. I've never done this before." The nurse was waiting for Dr. Lupo's arrival to check on my dilation status, but then she flashed a stern look of concern.

"We can't wait for Dr. Lupo. I need to check on you now," she insisted.

"When do I get the drugs for pain?" I panicked as the nurse examined me.

"You don't," she semi-shouted. "You're dilated to ten centimeters—this baby is ready to be born. Get a doctor in here, now!" The other nurse in the room ran out the door.

Dirk looked at me and said, "You'd better pick your favorite song because I don't think we'll listen to more than one."

I chose "More Than This." It seemed just right. I was so far beyond lonely drives around the lakes and complaining to Ida about my stalled life. What could ever be more than this?

A doctor appeared and said he'd assist me with Liza's birth. Dirk's face dropped. We didn't know this doctor from a man on the moon, and we trusted Dr. Lupo.

"Where is Dr. Lupo?" Dirk asked.

"Stuck in traffic," the doctor replied.

Two nurses instructed me on how to breathe my way through the pushing, and I received on-the-job training. The hypnotic Roxy Music song filled the room but failed to soothe me. As we had planned, Dirk attempted to ease the pain by squeezing my hand and reminding me to visualize peaceful places. As the labor pain twisted my insides, he encouraged me, "Go to the South of France! Go to the South of France!"

All I could do was focus inwardly on this pain and experience of birthing my baby. I looked at Dirk's sweet, earnest, about-to-become-a-dad face. He was trying to be so helpful, yet I snarled like a maniac who couldn't fathom what he was talking about. "There's *no way in hell* I am going to the South of France!"

57

Collapse

SUDDENLY, DR. LUPO RAN INTO THE ROOM WITH A BURST of energy and exclaimed, "Let's have this baby!" The other doctor quickly moved aside, and Dirk and I felt immense relief. We knew now, with Dr. Lupo in charge, it'd be all right.

Liza popped right out, Dirk cut the cord with a big grin on his face, and Dr. Lupo threw Liza on top of me like a hot potato. *Excuse me. Shouldn't we treat this tiny thing gently?* But there she was, this fresh little human, right there on my stomach. She was crying and coated with stuff—the most beautiful little girl.

What a wonder.

What a wonderful world.

"She looks so big," I said. She was just over four pounds, but it was the healthiest little four-pound package I'd ever laid my eyes on. A team of people swarmed in and whisked Liza to the NICU. Dirk went with them, and I fell back into the pillows with a massive smile on my face.

Dr. Lupo told me she'd raced through the snowstorm and run straight into the room to deliver Liza. "This is the first delivery I've ever done in my Eddie Bauer boots!" I exuded happiness. I couldn't believe I'd given birth to our little girl within one quick hour in the hospital.

"That went really well, Jennifer. You could do this again," Dr. Lupo said. Although she extended the idea that more children were possible, I didn't linger on that comment; it seemed too far beyond the moment I was in.

Immediately dialing my mom after Dr. Lupo left the room, I exclaimed, "I did it! I had the baby."

"What?" She was confused. "That's not funny."

"It's not funny because I'm not kidding," I said. "Liza was born."

"Are you serious?"

"Yes! I'm serious. Born in an hour. It went really fast."

"Oh my God. Larry!" she screamed to my dad in the background. "Jennifer had the baby!" And then back to me, "We're on our way!"

Dirk came back and wheeled me over to NICU to see our little one. Liza rested in an incubator. Nurses attached her to feeding tubes, oxygen tubes, and heart monitors.

I leaned over her Isolette, a plastic box of safety, and took in the marvel of her tiny body. Her delicate rosebud lips, the purple veins right beneath her translucent skin, and her shockingly long eyelashes wowed me.

Then I sang "The Ash Grove" softly. Her little head turned toward my song. *She knows me!* I don't remember being afraid of her fragility. I just remember soul-stirring exhilaration. How damaged could I be if I created a human?

But then I left the hospital, and Liza stayed. As if I'd left an arm behind, a piece of me seemed missing, an essential new extension of my life. I woke up each morning frantic and empty. I had to get to the hospital right away for my girl.

The nurses told us she'd stay in the NICU for about a week.

Like many other things, how quickly it became routine: a quick shower, throw on some clothes, drive downtown to the Hennepin County Medical Center (HCMC), race to the NICU, scrub my hands meticulously, cover my clothes with a hospital gown, and rush to the side of the Isolette where my daughter lay.

"Hi, peanut! Hey, it's your mom," I said to her ruddy little face covered in adhesive strips that held oxygen tubing to her face. "Lizabella, sweet pea, it's another good day. Did you grow for me last night? Did you remember to breathe?" I'd reach through the side porthole, grasp a miniature finger, and talk and sing and talk and sing, and absorb every bit of her.

A nurse named Mary Ann was in charge. She provided updates on how much Liza drank from a tiny bottle, breathing reports, apnea alerts, and how they monitored the monitors.

Dirk and I crooned over Liza. It's funny now when I think of showing off those newborn Polaroids with bursting pride. I remember a few sideways glances replaced the more typical "Oh, so cute" comments. Thank goodness nobody said, "Your baby looks like a starving bird." But I wonder if the thought had crossed a few minds. It wasn't until many years later when I looked again at those pictures that revealed the tender prematurity of my daughter after her birth.

I continued with my routine morning NICU visits, and Dirk and I visited together in the evening and on weekends. I fell back into a state of equilibrium, but I had no idea how quickly that would flip to chaos in the days ahead.

A week went by. The nurses said it would be another week. And another week. It became an agonizing week-by-week pronouncement of Liza's eventual discharge and ability to come home. It always seemed homecoming was right around the corner, just a little more, just a little more.

After three weeks, my doctor told me to check my creatinine to measure my kidney function. The result? My kidney was spilling additional protein. Dr. Somermeyer ordered an immediate ultrasound. It turned out that after the twenty-eight-week mark (when I learned about the kink in the ureter), the kink had worsened. Pressure from the backed-up fluid had damaged my kidney.

So while Liza stayed in the NICU at Hennepin County Medical Center, I headed to the University of Minnesota Medical Center for a drainage tube to bypass the kink. The upshot was I would sport an external bag—a temporary bladder—attached with Velcro around my leg and tucked under my pants. Not a typical young mom accessory, but a necessary one. Hopefully, the kink would straighten after my body resumed a nonpregnant state.

Mom brought me to the hospital, and we sat together in a room while a nurse checked me in. He asked all the same questions I'd heard a thousand times before. I gave all the same answers I'd said a thousand times before. Until he asked, "Did you just have a baby?" That was a new one.

"I did. My daughter, Liza, she's in NICU at Hennepin County. I'm anxious to get back to her."

"Oh, you look so cute for just having a baby!" he exclaimed. "Look at your little body." My mom rolled her eyes. She didn't find it necessary for him to comment on my "little body." Agreed, but he seemed playful, like a supportive cheerleader saying, "Girl, you look good."

"This shouldn't take long," he said. "They do these all the time. You'll be out of here quickly."

A doctor performed the procedure in the radiology department. I swallowed an antibiotic pill, and a nurse gave me a mild sedative. Then I fell into a haze and don't remember the radiologist placing the tube. Soon after, I awoke, and a nurse wheeled me back to the hospital room. When the drowsiness-inducing medications wore off, I'd be ready to go.

I put my clothes on and reclined in the bed while my mom sat in the corner chair. A nauseous wave washed over me. Dirk walked into the room. "How do you feel?" he asked.

A violent queasiness struck. "Not good." I fumbled for the

plastic puke container on top of the bedside table, pulling it toward me just in time. "I have to go to the bathroom," I said. "It's urgent." I jumped out of bed and collapsed on the floor.

"*Nurse!*" Dirk yelled.

My mom shot up from that corner chair, ran out into the hall, and screamed, "We need a doctor in the room!"

A passing nurse snidely replied, "Well, we've got plenty of those around here." My panicked mom later told me she had wanted to deck her. Dirk peeled me off the floor and helped get me back to the bed. Another nurse raced in and immediately saw I was in distress. She fetched a bed pan and took my blood pressure. I remember hearing it was 55/30. I saw the eyes in the room widen with concern, while everything inside me wanted to come out.

We learned infected urine had backed up into my kidney. When the doctor placed the tube, the infection spread throughout my bloodstream, causing sepsis, a dangerous blood infection.

My blood poisoned me as the bacteria raged. Nurses swiftly moved me to the ICU and flooded my system with antibiotics. The goal: to restore my blood pressure and keep my organs functioning. All the while, my fragile baby girl was at another hospital in the NICU.

I was too out of it to grasp the immensity of the experience. It exists now like a blurry image with soft edges—a dream I try to piece together with snippets of memory. Mom came and went. Dirk gave me updates on Liza. Post-pregnancy bleeding all over the bed. Grogginess. Comprehensive body aches for my girl.

A nurse with a tight ponytail and pinched expression cared for me in the ICU. She couldn't leave my side because of my condition. While checking continuous blood pressure readings, she kept a steady stream of antibiotics flowing to battle a bacteria war. After the sheets revealed a bloody I-just-had-a-baby mess, her words dried up. I imagined she wasn't loving her shift with me, but her disinterest and the stained sheets were the least of my concerns. I longed for privacy so I could sob because *oh my God, what's happening?*

It wasn't my health I worried about; it was Liza's. My daughter was my priority, and I wouldn't let my nurse disregard me as some high-risk thirty-one-year-old woman in ICU. She didn't realize who she was dealing with. I was a survivor, and all I wanted to think about was Liza's apnea monitor and if she sucked and swallowed correctly. Was she breathing without interruption? I yearned to hold her.

After five days of massive antibiotic IVs, I stabilized and moved out of that purgatory-like ICU space. The infection cleared. I showered and slowly put on my clothes, a return to my regular, albeit shaky, self. We received discharge orders, and Dirk and I returned home. Exhausted. Shaken to my core. But determined. Because I was a mom now, and I had a very important job to do.

58

Frantic

I WAS FRANTIC TO SEE LIZA, BUT WE COULDN'T VISIT THE NICU until the next morning. Our favorite nurse, Mary Ann, had been caring for her all week. In an emotional state, at home in bed, I bemoaned, "What if Liza loves Mary Ann and doesn't love me?"

Dirk assured me, "Probably not likely that after you raise her, she'll tell people, 'I love my mom, but the thing is, when I was a few weeks old, there was this special nurse . . .'"

I wasn't convinced. "These early weeks are so important." He hugged me and smiled. Clearly, he didn't buy into my concerns. My return hug was limp and floppy. The infection saga had taken a toll, and as I snuggled up to Dirk, trying to put it all behind me, shards of trauma lodged within me like dispersed bullet fragments. I felt as solid as steam. *Please don't let me evaporate from this world.* I held on to my husband, hoping he'd contain me.

Sepsis can kill people, but I couldn't linger on that fact. I tossed aside the thoughts of how close I had come to dying. All that mattered was that I got better. And I wanted to comfort Dirk—what an ordeal he'd just been through. He bore the brunt of it, really, because I'd existed in a fog while he traveled between two hospitals with the worst outcomes running through his mind. *What if she doesn't make it? Is my daughter going to grow up without her mother?* How did he appear so stoic and unruffled through that?

I assumed he'd held it together for me. Surely, he must have fallen apart somewhere. Maybe at night he'd shed tears in bed, or in the shower, or on the drive between hospitals. Later, I asked him, and he said he'd flipped on his crisis management switch. Fueled by adrenaline, he'd remained focused on each moment that led to the next. Visit me. Visit Liza. Go home and feed the dog. Shovel the eight inches of snow that had accumulated from the winter storms. Back to visit me. Back to Liza.

It would take three years before his fears rose from the deep like a submarine.

Yet now here we were together, meshed in exhaustion and relief on the edge of much-needed sleep. The next morning, we quickly showered and dressed, gulped coffee, and headed out to see our baby girl together. I rushed through the obligatory handwashing and hospital gown procedure and burst through the double doors into the preemie unit. The antiseptic smell in this space resembled the odorous assault in the ICU—yet this air smelled sweeter knowing it circulated around my girl.

There she was, my precious peanut, in her Isolette. "Liza, it's your mom. I missed you so much," I said as tears filled my eyes. I sang "The Ash Grove" and lifted my baby to cuddle her snugly in my arms. Her delicate body generated heat like a tiny furnace. Audibly, I released a breath to exhale the chaos of the previous seven days. I watched the rise and fall of her small chest and cherished her healthy, developed lungs. I wanted to occupy this moment of peace forever.

Dirk smiled at us, and his eyes welled over. With his face close to hers, he said, "Your mom's here, little sweetheart; your mom's here."

59

Snip

NOT LONG AFTER WE BROUGHT LIZA HOME, DIRK TOLD me that pregnancy was something he could endure one time and one time only. "We're so lucky to have one beautiful daughter," he said. "I will not go through this ever again." He then quickly scheduled a vasectomy, and snip . . . our family was complete.

Dr. Lupo had tossed out her "you can do it again" notion before I almost lost my life from sepsis. After what we'd just gone through, I feared another pregnancy too and didn't question Dirk's unilateral decision. More pregnancies were not meant to be. But three makes a family, and I felt wildly lucky.

Feed, sleep, and grow. That was the task for Liza's first several months at home. We kept a careful watch on her breathing with the monitors, while a home health nurse came and checked her weekly weight gain. Preemies, because of their immature immune systems, are at extra risk of contracting RSV, a respiratory infection. So the doctors told us to keep Liza indoors until April. By then the infection risk would be reduced, and she'd be stronger.

In the fall before Liza was born, I'd planted tulip bulbs in the landscaped area by our front door. I waited with anticipation for their white-and-pink petals to bloom with pops of yellow in the center. My Liza tulips. When those petals bloomed in the late spring, I could safely stroll her around the block.

I snuggled in with my baby, worked from home, and received many visits from my mom and friends. Meanwhile, I still had a kink in my ureter and ingested daily antibiotics to keep infections at bay. My doctor kept a close eye on my kidney function, and my health uncertainty hung in the air like humidity.

Liza, like all babies, was an exhausting little bundle. It took six months before she slept through the night. She cried for a bottle every three hours (medications prevented me from breast-feeding), and Dirk and I took turns with the 1:00 a.m. and 4:00 a.m. feedings. It was easier for me because I would wake up, feed her in my arms on the love seat in her peaceful, pink-walled room, and fall back asleep.

Dirk never fell back asleep, so he'd wake up and stay up. Sleep deprivation made him a little (a lot) crabby. One evening, he told me the exhaustion was compromising his work.

"How so?" I asked as I held Liza.

"I've got patients talking about their problems," he explained, "and I pinch myself—hard—so I don't nod off."

"It's never a good therapy session when your psychologist snores," I replied.

"I actually restrain myself from saying, 'You think *you've* got problems? I haven't slept for six months!'"

"Yeah, don't do that," I said, and laughed. But he didn't. Too exhausted. Our pediatrician finally said Liza had put on enough weight, so she didn't need feedings as frequently through the night, and he cautioned we should expect her to cry. Then our doctor described the Ferber method—a systematic approach to train a baby to soothe themselves back to sleep. Dirk and I bit our fingernails through increasingly extended periods of baby howling before entering her room. And when we stepped in at the appropriate interval, we couldn't comfort her with touch. Basically, it's cruel and unusual punishment for both parents and babies.

But Ferberize we did. Liza's habitual (but unnecessary) feeding time came. She wailed. We cringed and waited. On the first night, Dirk and I held off for three minutes before we tiptoed into her room. Over two days, we'd stretched it to five. The intervals increased. She kept crying, and the long spans broke my heart. I wanted to cry too. (Dirk wanted to sleep.)

As the process continued, we worked up to seventeen minutes of wailing endurance. And I couldn't take it anymore. The poor thing. Dirk urged me to hold back, but I rushed to her door. Hand on the knob. And right then, in a magical instant . . . she stopped. After seventeen minutes of piercing screams on the fifth night, she stopped crying. And guess what? She slept through the night peacefully from that point on.

It was another lesson in the elusive quality of time. During those moments, Liza's sleeping ability seemed the biggest thing in the world. She's in her twenties now. I've got to say, she's a great sleeper, and I don't worry about it one bit.

Winter came and went. Liza ate, slept, and grew. Spring arrived, as it always does. As if on cue, those delicate, resilient tulips punched through the soil after the long cold season. I strolled Liza through the neighborhood with an uncontained grin. How heartening and familiar to experience determined tulips mustering the resilience to bloom again. They survive through the most brutal of winters. And so do we.

60.

Stay Here

TWO MONTHS LATER, WHEN LIZA WAS EIGHT MONTHS old, my doctor declared that surgery was the only permanent solution to fix the kink caused by my pregnancy. Another surgery awaited.

Dirk's mom and dad visited from Pennsylvania to help Dirk while I stayed in the hospital. We set Merv and Arlene up in our basement, the only space we had to accommodate them. They were gracious and never complained about their fold-out bed in the cold room downstairs. And Arlene adored spending time with her newest granddaughter in Minnesota.

Dirk's mom insisted on taking Liza from me at every turn. As I would give Liza a bottle, Arlene would bound around the corner and chirp, "Oh, let me do it!" But I clung to every second I could spend with Liza before my surgery departure.

"I want to do it," I said, tamping back tears. Arlene didn't understand (since I was a seasoned pro at having surgery) that this operation swathed me in dread. My previous sepsis scare reverberated in my soul. The lingering aftershocks left me hyper-aware that things can go wrong.

What if I go to the hospital and I don't come back? I can't abandon Liza. Who will help her with her homework? Who will she run to when she falls down and needs a kiss to make it all better? Who will care whether she eats nutritious food and who will help her draw fancy pictures and throw balls and create books and pull her hair into a ponytail and tell her teachers she is a smart kid and stick up for her when someone is mean and let her know she's a miracle and the most special kid in the world? Please let me raise her. Please let me be here.

Dirk and I were supposed to be partners in parenthood. He couldn't navigate babysitters, mean girls, and Liza's first period without me. And how would he tell her what a wonderful mother I'd been if I never got the chance to prove it? What kind of therapy would be adequate for the future woman version of our daughter if she lost her mom at eight months old? This upcoming surgery broke me open. I'd learned to face a lot of health scares and accept my life one day at a time. But not this. I couldn't wrap my mind around not being Liza's mom.

My prayers revved up on overdrive. So I resorted to what I'd done for the previous eight years. I visualized being okay. I played this movie over and over in my mind—returning home, holding Liza, giving her a bottle, and wrapping her in my arms.

The next morning, Dirk popped in while I held Liza in bed. "Get up, Jen. We should leave in an hour." He walked over and kissed my cheek. Liza's face lit up with smiles of wonder, and she grabbed my nose.

"Let me take her," Dirk said. "You get ready." Sitting up, I extended my arms, wanting her back.

Before departing, I hugged Dirk's parents first. When I held Liza's tiny burrito-wrapped body, which nestled so perfectly in my arms, I kissed her goodbye and transformed into a tear-producing machine. Dissolving in front of my in-laws embarrassed me, but I couldn't stop. This would be the first operation with full anesthesia I'd undergo as a mom. And that made all the difference. The stakes seemed so much higher, so my previous pre-surgery calming mantra, *You don't have to do anything; just go in and go to sleep,* failed to soothe me.

Time to go.

In the cold pre-op room, flat on my back, my muscles stiffened from distress. And my mind, refusing my positive visualizations, crafted sorrow-filled narratives of leaving my baby daughter alone.

A sleep-inducing injection and backwards countdown pulled me from my awareness. When I woke in a drowsy, medicated stupor five hours later, euphoric relief overwhelmed me. My nurse explained it had been a long and complicated procedure. But the skillful work of my surgeon, Dr. Gruesner, cleared the way for my kidney to continue doing its job. *I am awake! I am alive!* I knew then I would return to Liza and fulfill *my* job. As a mom.

After three days in the hospital, I returned home and nestled Liza protectively against my heart. Happy tears flooded my cheeks as I recited *thank you, thank you, thank you* to the powers that be. I would move forward, stay alive, and raise my daughter.

61

Drift

TWO AND A HALF YEARS LATER, MY CUDDLY BABY HAD transformed into a busy toddler—a little being who claimed a lot of space. Fake food, a red cash register, scattered piles of plastic money, and an explosive collection of Polly Pockets (tiny plastic dolls I called "the little guys") accessorized our family room. As a three-year-old, Liza favored anything pink and purple, including feather boas and metallic hats. What fun is it to be three if you can't parade around in Liberace-style outfits?

When she acted out in disequilibrium as toddlers do (once she threw a small red truck at my head), I turned to my library of how-to-be-a-parent books. Dr. Brazelton to the rescue. Sometimes I gave her a time-out. Sometimes I gave myself a time-out. Even during occasional tantrums that made me want to scream, I remembered the luckiness of her.

She attended a preschool close to my office, where I had become the vice president of sales and marketing for the family company. It was a big title for a small business, but I continued to work with a steady stream of fascinating clients to help them plan their unique homes. Our clients' elaborate dreams included rock climbing walls, basketball courts, gift-wrapping rooms, indoor pools, and outdoor kitchens. I enjoyed learning about my clients' hobbies and habits to create spaces to nurture their lives.

My work arrangement allowed me to pick Liza up at preschool each day at 3:30. At the day's end, Dirk arrived home, and I'd carry on about some amusing exchange with a client or Liza's signs of genius (like a masterpiece drawing of an elongated triangle lady with a pinhead). The marker dexterity!

"What's new with you?" I'd ask Dirk, prodding unsuccessfully for a willing conversation partner.

But gradually, while Liza and my work thrived, Dirk and I drifted apart. He was busy with his practice and highly stressed. Obviously, there's little comparison between the gravity of working with mentally ill patients and custom home clients. But he'd become quiet, and his disconnection worried me. He retreated like he'd done before we got married. But at that time, he'd pondered the monumental decision of marriage. So why now? I resorted to my go-to assumption—the destruction of my disease had spread to our marriage. *What if Dirk can't handle my medical mess anymore?*

Then I stuffed down my concerns. *Don't ruffle feathers. Be easy.* So I waited a long time to voice my worries. Finally, one evening after dinner, I interrupted Dirk's intense laptop focus and said, "I think we need to connect more; I don't feel like things are okay with us."

"We'll do more," he said, without lifting his eyes from the screen. We perched together on the same sofa, but I stared at the television, and he stared at his computer. Physically close. Emotionally distant. Was my "bother" too much? The horror of the unforeseen sepsis three years earlier, the premature birth, and my surgery when Liza was eight months old? Maybe this heavy load tipped the scales, resulting in a weight he couldn't carry.

My thoughts festered. *Maybe he should have listened to his mom's concerns.* Like the emotional equivalent of a jack-in-the-box, the thought popped up, and I pushed it back under the lid that concealed it. And again, pop. *I may be too damaged for this marriage.*

62

Thick Air

I DOGGEDLY MANAGED MY HEALTH, SWALLOWED TWENTY
pills a day, and attended my required doctors' visits. One of the
more troublesome side effects of autoimmune medication is skin
cancer. Every month, my dermatologist scrutinized my skin
through a magnifying glass.

If Dr. Tope had had a frequent-flier program, I would've
racked up a lot of miles.

Compared to the general population, transplant patients
experience a higher risk of squamous cell carcinoma (SCC).
Most SCCs are slow growers, but a compromised immune system can propel these lesions to spread rapidly. As in most things,
early detection is the key. Diligent dermatology, gobs of daily
sunscreen, and limited sun exposure comprised my routine.

I got used to this aspect of my transplant life and tossed the
word *cancer* around lightly. "Hey Dirk, got some cancers cut out
today," I'd tell him, as if I'd had my split ends trimmed. "How're
you doing?" I didn't assign the same gravity to some of my issues
as Dirk did; we each had different force fields of energy around
my health. In time his energy felt like an emotional barricade.

Increasingly frustrated, I brought it up again. "I think we
need to talk more," I said one night after a long day. We sat in
bed, pajamas on, television humming, while Liza slept soundly
in her pink-walled room. I hoped to improve things between us,
but I also shrunk away from voicing my concern. Had I become
the dreaded burden that I feared?

"It's not a good time for me now. I'm really busy at work." I thought his answer revealed something blatant about his priorities. *You don't have time to discuss your marriage because you are too busy at work? Maybe that's the problem here.* These thoughts stayed inside my head. "Well, just so you know, I'm unraveling." These words came out of my mouth.

Then I vacillated between spirited (*I'm actually a fabulous wife*) and pissed off (*If work stresses you out, at least talk to me about it*). But these were additional conversations I had with myself. Go figure. *I* didn't want to talk too much about how *he* didn't talk. I was the pot. He was the black kettle.

I tucked these thoughts into my arsenal of grievances and thought Dirk seemed like a roommate version of a husband. And a lousy roommate at that.

One evening, I met girlfriends at an Italian restaurant in the Uptown area of Minneapolis. Dirk was working late, and my mom, now also known as Grammy, played with Liza. My friend Carrie poured us a glass of wine from the bottle on the table and took a sip. "I hate this wine," she said.

Without skipping a beat, I said, "I hate Dirk." Oops, Freudian slip. I vented, and we talked about how marriage is hard, communication is work, and becoming parents changes everything. Normal ebbs and flows. But I knew there was a reckoning to come.

Dirk didn't get the clue that I was approaching the end of my proverbial rope. When we traveled through the airport, I heard the announcement, "Caution, you are nearing the end of the moving walkway," speak directly to me. *Caution, you are nearing the end of your flipping rope.* I looked at Dirk as if the overhead lady's voice revealed my inner thoughts. I wanted to say, "Did you hear that?!"

It didn't help that my kidney was in a state of gradual decline, as expected, and my creatinine kept steadily rising. My last transplant had taken place five years earlier, so we knew what waited in the wings in the years ahead.

I felt pathetic. People in this world suffer true hardships. How dare I question this marriage. Wasn't this everything I'd hoped for? I tried to tap into a positive perspective, but this wasn't an issue my mind power could solve alone. Silent tensions thickened the air between us, and I'd learned all too well from autoimmunity—unseen things can cause destruction.

We'd said goodbye to the 1990s, and the year 2000 was upon us. The dot-com technology bubble burst, Bill Clinton stepped aside for George Bush after we learned of hanging chads, and *American Beauty* won five Academy Awards. In the almost seven years since we'd tied the knot in 1994 (you know what they say about seven years), I'd become professionally and maternally validated, yet I felt barricaded from the love of my husband. Jerk.

Except—Dirk was not a full-time jerk. Here was a guy who saved lives for a living, a guy who'd drop anything for a friend, a guy who was protective, open to self-improvement, and a generous tipper. So why this? Why now? I quickly rekindled the idea I'd be better off to pack up my damaged self and be alone, free from outside forces that squashed my positivity.

Marriage is hard, and chronic illness adds a tricky layer. But chronic illness or not, the effort to make a marriage work applies to most couples. According to Dr. John Gottman, a renowned psychologist and marriage researcher, many couples drift apart within seven years. And 50 percent of marriages end within these seven years.

The problem, Gottman found, is that the average couple waits six years before seeking help. Things unsaid loosen the seams. Guilty. Dirk and I had loose seams.

One evening, we'd finished dinner and were loading the

dishwasher. The air around us felt stale and still. Our relationship distance had saddened me for months. Then Dirk announced he was ready to talk. Finally. I had begged for this, but now I didn't know if I could hear what he might say. We retreated to the family nook and sat face-to-face. His eyes opened wide, and he leaned toward me. He started, "That sepsis episode turned me upside down."

"It did me too," I said. I could feel my eyebrows lift as my eyes searched his. I'd wondered how he'd been so composed during that time. "What does that have to do with your silence? You've retreated." The desire to bolt ran through me as I awaited his answer. *Sit with this. Don't repel his words like Teflon. This is not a support group you can reject.*

"I know. I didn't do it consciously; I just feel overwhelmed sometimes. In a way, it seemed easier not to care." Oddly relieved, now I knew I wasn't crazy to think he was distant. I steadied myself to learn more, even as my heart pumped faster.

"What are you afraid of?" A lump rose in my throat, and I tried to swallow it down.

"Losing you. It all changed once we had Liza. I'm scared of the future for her. And me. What if the worst happens and you die? When I think of that, I shut down. I didn't want to feel anything."

I didn't know what to say. I mean, I got it on one level. But then it made me mad. *Let me get this straight*, I thought. *You shut me out because I was the source of your potential future pain?* I tried to let that settle, but it seemed mean to leave me dangling alone while we were supposed to be together. Suffice it to say, we had some untangling to do. "Well, that's painfully honest," I said, breaking eye contact and clutching myself with tight elbows. In a quiet voice, I continued, "If we can't have an attentive, loving marriage, I want something else."

Dirk recoiled like I'd punched him in the face. His eyes broadcast vulnerability like the night he'd proposed.

"I know I held back on honest conversations," I admitted. "But I'm trying to stay positive. When you're down, I must be up. We're like a teeter-totter. We need to balance." Wasn't it my job to keep us upbeat, ignore that terrorist in the attic, and paint our lives with broad strokes of optimism?

"No, Jen. No. You don't need to balance my emotions with positivity. We need to talk about the shitty parts."

"But what if I want to rise above the shitty parts?" My face reddened. "This is how I make it okay!" I blurted out. "Why is that a *bad* thing?" I felt myself coming undone.

"You're so good at making it okay," he said soothingly. "But you don't need to edit my emotions. And it's okay to feel *everything*. Optimism isn't an emotion."

Maybe my radical positivity and creative denial were not always beneficial. Did Dirk have a point? Was I stifling his ability to be honest? Maybe I suffocated *my* ability to be honest too. Perfectionism failure. If lovability motivated my quest to be "perfect," that backfired. It was equivalent to building a moat when I needed a bridge.

After we dedicated ourselves to figuring it out, we put in the work and achieved clarity on what was happening. Our dueling techniques of coping had clashed—I ramped up my make-it-okayness while he withdrew. In alternate ways, we each held emotional shields of self-protection for survival.

I remembered how unburdened I'd felt after I opened up to the priest in the hospital. Then I considered how essential my unvarnished relationship was with my mom. So now I had to be wholly authentic with Dirk. And he with me.

An emotional window opened, and fresh air circulated around us. The energy in our house lightened, and Dirk emerged with a new vitality. Honest communication stitched us back together.

Thank goodness we became whole again. Because two years later, in July 2002, our terrorist paid a visit. We united with shared strength to muscle through my third transplant. And a very special transplant it was. Unlike the first two, I didn't wait on the donor list. Unlike the first two, I didn't start dialysis beforehand. And unlike the first two, a living donor stepped in.

Since my first transplant in 1990, developments in antigen matching had changed significantly. So what had been unfeasible became possible. Wondrously, at sixty-five years old, my dear mom became a suitable match to donate her kidney to me, after all.

63

Dog Down

I RECEIVED MOM'S KIDNEY IN THE SUMMER BEFORE
Liza started kindergarten, and she gifted me time and energy to
relish more morsels of regular life. I volunteered twice a week at
Liza's school, launched into impromptu dance contests at home,
found passion in my work, and golfed badly with my husband.

What can I say about my mom? Kidney donation or not, she
is like oxygen to me. Appreciative sentences about her are just
the iceberg's tip of deep gratitude.

In 2005, three years after my mom's gift, Dirk and I sold our
house. We had purchased a lot and contracted with my dad's
company to build a new home in a kid-friendly neighborhood.
While construction was underway, we lived in a big-windowed,
sun-filled apartment across from Lake Calhoun. Our temporary
digs flanked the Parkway where Dirk and I had first met. We'd
come a long way since then.

I hit the milestone of forty. Dirk's practice had grown significantly, and we were parenting a spunky kid. Zoe, no longer a
wild puppy, had mellowed into a relatively calm dog over the
past ten years. And life changed for her on the twenty-second
floor of our cramped apartment. She couldn't sniff around at
leisure anymore in our previous home's fenced yard, and I noticed a drop in her playful energy.

In the spring, on a Saturday afternoon, Liza, her friend
Franny, and I went across the street to the lakeside park. The

girls bolted to the swing set. A cloudless powder-blue sky met the darker blue water, dotted by white sails and swimmers. Runners, walkers, tail-wagging dogs and their owners circled the lake.

Zoe ambled slowly, sniffing every blade of grass. When she suddenly toppled over, I thought she'd tripped. "Get up, silly Zoe," I said. She tried but couldn't do it.

A nearby woman rushed over. "I saw your dog go down. Can I help you? I work with animals."

"I don't know what happened," I said rapidly, dazed with confusion. I felt my eyes expand as I stared at this kind woman, begging her to do something.

She crouched down, listened to Zoe's breathing, and felt for her heartbeat. "Your dog is in distress. You need to get her to a vet right away." My heart pounded as I looked at poor Zoe lying on her side in the grass, one brown eye gazing at me as if to say, *Help me.* Liza and Franny ran over to see what was happening.

I punched Dirk's number into the phone. Frantically, I blurted out that Zoe had collapsed. "I need help! Zoe's not right, and we need to take her to the vet."

Moments later, Dirk ran over from the apartment and lifted Zoe in his arms. He rushed back across the street, holding her, and turned to say, "Take your car and meet me."

Liza and I dropped Franny at her nearby home and raced to the emergency animal hospital. As we pulled into the parking lot, Dirk walked slowly toward us. The corners of his mouth curved downward; his face said it all. I let out a gasp and steadily pounded on the steering wheel.

Liza watched me with enormous eyes. "What? What is it, Mom?"

"The look on his face—I don't like the look. I don't like the look on his face!" I stammered, my voice tight and high. Dirk approached with red-rimmed eyes, and I lowered the window.

"She's dying." Dirk's chin crumpled. "The vet said her heart is trying to stop. She's shutting down. Come in and see her."

I grabbed Liza's hand and the three of us walked swiftly inside, but it was too late. Zoe had died. In an instant, Zoe was no longer with us. I wanted to say goodbye. Dirk stayed with Liza while an assistant led me back to the room where Zoe lay. She looked like she was sleeping peacefully. I folded over her still body and told her what a great dog she was.

The eleven years we'd spent with Zoe replayed in my mind. Zoe had entered our lives as an adorable puppy when I started the second round of dialysis, and we'd lived together in our Golden Valley house before Liza materialized from my dream to my daughter. That sneaky thief, time, reared up like in that *Marley & Me* flashback scene where you think, *Where has all the time gone?* and then, *Where is it going?* and then, *Did we love her enough when she was here?* and finally, *Do we love each other enough?*

I cried for two days. Really. It surprised me too. We all know dogs come and go. Everybody has stories of dogs loved and dogs lost. Even so, I felt a profound slap from the passing of time and the cruelty of death.

It also scared me. I ruminated on the notion that my life, like Zoe's, like all of ours, would end one day, maybe without notice. I tapped into a deep place where my repressed fears were stored. Hot liquid thoughts gushed up like a geyser. I had made it to my forties, and the "die young" fears that Elliott expressed years ago had not come to be. But now, older, wiser, I was sure that death was the only absolute thing amongst all this uncertainty.

Liza had never known life without Zoe, but despite her sadness, she was remarkably wise. She tried to comfort *me*; my third grader gave me calming talks about "the circle of life." I marveled at her maturity about death and attempt to understand and articulate it. She wrote a poem about her loss, and her teacher, Mrs. Bartow, read it aloud to her class. It was a notable mom moment for me; I fell apart while my kid was strong.

I thought about Dirk's retreat years ago because he was afraid that love would lead to loss. Well, he was right, love leads to loss. So perhaps what it means to love a pet, and how hard it is to lose one, crystallizes so much of what life is—having the guts to love full force because the joy you gain is worth the pain.

Perhaps the inevitability of death is the best motivation for living a good life. Every day. Right now.

64.

Just Because

IN NOVEMBER 2006, OUR NEW HOUSE WAS COMPLETE. Mom's kidney worked like a champ. Mundane moments? Yes, please! Our home came to life with birthday bashes, holiday turkeys with all the fixings, fist-pumping (and on-the-feet cheering) for the Steelers and Vikings, giggly girl sleepovers, and pizza/karaoke parties with the best bad singing ever. (Aunt Lucy's version of Elvis's "Hound Dog," uniquely delivered as a talking rap, took the prize.) The only missing piece was Zoe.

The following spring, eleven-year-old Liza and I talked about getting another dog, but Dirk wasn't on board. He cited the work involved, the cost, and the responsibility. We didn't believe these were reasonable obstacles to loving a dog, so we persisted.

When Dirk was away on a business trip, Liza and I spent an evening researching various breeds. Just for fun. We came across adorable pictures of black-and-white dogs. Tibetan terriers. After reading about their lively, fun-loving temperament, we were intrigued. Our online search expanded to local breeders.

That's when I discovered that Zoe's breeder, Earl, besides breeding wheaten terriers, now bred Tibetans. Surely *that* was a sign, so I called him. Earl explained the differences between the two breeds and then dropped this on me: "We have some Tibetan puppies right now, and there's one left. He's a little guy, and we call him Flash. You should come and meet him."

"My husband is out of town, so I should probably wait," I said. I knew this idea pulled me into dangerous territory. Looking up puppies online and calling Earl was one thing. Going to *see* the pups with Liza? That was something else entirely.

"You don't have to do anything but meet him. Your daughter will have fun seeing the pups. Just come over and play." Yeah, right.

Like a sucker, I drove twenty minutes with Liza to see the cuddly cuties. When we got there, the most adorable black-and-white puppy bounded out the door. He jumped on Liza and showered her with sweet puppy kisses.

No surprise, Liza fell in love at first sight. Yes, me too. We played for a while and left with aching hearts and a firm conviction we'd met *the* dog destined to be ours. Liza called Dirk and told him about little Flash. "Please, Dad! PLEASE! I *already* love him!" Even though I wasn't on the line, I could hear his frustrated sigh.

When Dirk was back in town, we all took the trek to see little Flash. Liza bubbled with excitement in the back seat. Dirk's eyebrows and lips tightened as he leaned toward me and asked, "Is there really a choice here?"

"There is," I said. "Your choice is to love Flash too." I smiled and gave him a nudge.

"Dad, he's so cute. Just wait," Liza told him. Again, Flash bounded out the door and Liza unleashed infectious giggles. I wouldn't say Dirk fell in love (he didn't), but he agreed (reluctantly) that we could bring little Flash home. What dad could resist brown-eyed pleas from his daughter? Besides, she was an only child; the kid needed a dog, right?

With Flash on her lap on the way home, Liza nestled her face against his fur and cooed. Dirk gripped the wheel like a vise and stared straight ahead. Liza ran through a million ideas for puppy names, and finally announced that Timmy, the Tibetan terrier, was the chosen name of our new four-legged family member.

It occurred to me that a new dog had joined our lives each time I started dialysis. Mickey, my parents' dog, had folded in way back when Nick visited me from Seattle and dialysis was brand-new. Next, Dirk and I adopted Zoe when dialysis round two began. I hoped Timmy wasn't an omen. I allowed the thought in and let it out—Timmy's acquisition had nothing to do with kidney failure or recruiting a pet to ease a difficult time.

Instead, cute Timmy entered our lives, at the insistence of my daughter and me, to add joy. And that seemed a perfectly wonderful reason. Just like my parents' long-ago ice cream outings hadn't hinged upon report card performance, adopting our loveable thirteen-pounder didn't hinge on declining health. This dog, Timmy, exemplified ordinary people getting a dog to love. Just because.

65

Small Giant

IN 2009, THREE YEARS AFTER TIMMY JOINED US, the holidays approached, and so did my parents' fiftieth anniversary. Party planning was underway to celebrate this milestone. Now forty-six years old, Steve was still a New York bachelor, and his hope for marriage by thirty-five (expressed many years ago) had passed.

Mixed into conversations about the guest list and menu, Steve mentioned his recent travels to South America. The highlight of his trip had occurred in Cartagena, Colombia. Her name was Merly.

"We had an amazing time," he said. I could hear the buoyancy in his voice. His words smiled. "I hardly speak Spanish, but it was an electric connection." Merly and Steve had maintained a long-distance relationship from the moment he left.

"So, are you in love with her?" I asked, sensing his sparkling energy.

"I'd say that. Yeah. We're in love." This was big news. And I couldn't wait to meet Merly. She'd applied for a tourist visa and awaited its approval.

We set a December party date, and Dirk and I hosted the event. Steve flew in from New York. Aunt Lucy, other aunts, uncles, cousins, nieces, nephews, and all those special people woven into my parents' lives showed up. My mom's hair (compliments of her hair stylist) was still strawberry blond, and her fair, soft skin revealed gentle lines of wisdom. She'd recovered well after our surgeries seven and a half years earlier. And it floored me how fast that time had gone. I could hear the clock ticking.

Trim and dazzling, my mom stood by my dad's side, whose full head of coarse dark hair had whitened around his temples. Conversations and laughter melded with Frank Sinatra–style big band music. Dirk quieted the crowd, Steve dimmed the lights, and I gave a tribute. I asked the guests to imagine hitting a fifty-year rewind button. Dwight D. Eisenhower was the president, *Ben-Hur* was the top film, and a young teacher named Liz fell in love with a mortgage banker named Larry.

I took in the synchronized clinking of the glasses held high, and Dirk put his arm around me. As we smiled with my parents, I appreciated the anniversaries I'd shared with Dirk. We stood side by side, toasting my parents' milestone, and again, it struck me . . . what a wonderful world.

Meanwhile, I knew Steve had Merly on his mind. I looked at him talking to an old buddy of Dad's and noticed how his shoulders relaxed and his eyes shined. Was he thinking about marriage as he celebrated our parents' milestone? He placed his arm around my mom, and she rested her head on his shoulder.

More toasts. Stories told of cherished family holidays. We recounted the many perfectly cooked turkeys (brine it, that's the secret) and Dad's gourmet stuffing, which includes a surprise ingredient each time. (*Are those apricots?*) We reminisced about a frazzled holiday, when powdered sugar thickened the gravy instead of flour, the oven conked out, and the green beans fell on the floor. Aunt Lucy came into the kitchen to assist Mom. At the end of her rope, Mom snarled at her sister, "Tell them the goddamn dinner is ready."

Aunt Lucy, as told, marched into the living room where everyone engaged in carefree belly laughs, political debates, and libations. "Excuse me," she said, to quiet the family. Then, enunciating slowly and theatrically, she stated, "Liz wants you to know the goddamn dinner is ready." We have referred to our holiday meals as the "goddamn dinner" ever since.

We laugh about it still because we've learned, in the middle of chaos, when tightly planned events become a circus, it's the people that make the moment fun. This crowd bound together with memories in joyful celebration of my parents.

Despite the energetic camaraderie, I fought exhaustion. With puffy eyes, I looked down at the noticeable swelling pooled in my ankles and on the tops of my feet. Amid the noisy, affectionate banter, I drew in a sharp breath. I knew exactly what was going on.

Here we go again.

Although it seemed like yesterday, it'd been almost eight years since Mom and I sipped coffee at her kitchen table and she'd insisted on giving me her kidney. "I want to do this!" she'd said.

I'd pulled back with hesitation, "Mom . . ."

She interrupted and looked at me straight on. "One question. Would you do this for Liza?" She left no space for an answer and said, "I'm doing this. Don't say another word." She knew I'd do anything for Liza. Mom must have seen a flash in my eyes because she looked satisfied—as if she'd clarified something essential that she wanted me to realize—*you* are *my* daughter.

When I was a young girl, Mom had sat with me in that same spot and nursed my don't-feel-goods with cinnamon toast and 7-Up. There was healing power in her buttered bread sprinkled with the perfect ratio of sugar and spice. She transferred her love through that toast, and it always made me feel better. As moms do, she'd always been by my side trying to make everything okay.

My mom's maternal force made me think of Liza's precarious start as a preemie. Apnea, breathing monitors, tiny bottles, the transition to baby food. Naptimes ferociously guarded, the car seat fastened tight, limits on *Clifford the Big Red Dog*. Fresh air. The worship of her bedtime routine. A conversation during her nightly tuck-in when she was a toddler came to mind. She'd said, "Mom, you're like my garbage man."

"Why's that, honey?" I'd asked, pulling her covers snug around her.

"Because when I tell you scary thoughts, you take them away." Her eyes widened as her little hands gripped the satin edge of the chenille blanket by her face.

"I will always take away your garbage thoughts," I'd replied, and kissed her good night. Isn't that what moms are hardwired to do? Clean it up. Make it better. As she had done for years, my mom was attempting to take away my garbage. On a very grand scale.

Despite my reluctance, Mom hadn't taken no for an answer. She knew she only needed one of her two kidneys, and she wanted to save me from dialysis and a lengthy, uncertain wait on the transplant list. (A five-year wait was typical.) The wait is long because of supply and demand—more people need a kidney than there are kidneys available.

In 2022, according to Donate Life America, over one hundred thousand people were awaiting a kidney transplant. And each day, seventeen people die waiting. That's why living donors like my mom are remarkable and benevolent problem solvers.

Thank you, Mom.

Thank you. Thank you. Thank you.

I remembered when my mother-in-law had said, "You don't know this because you are not a mother, but when your child hurts, you hurt." Maybe she'd been thinking about my mom when she said this. And now that I was a mom, I understood the truth in her words. It saddened me to think of the pain that had broadsided my mom after we first strapped into our medical roller-coaster ride.

When I had been diagnosed years earlier and returned home, loads of infections and fevers cropped up. So my mom set up pots and pans on the floor by my bed. It was her unconventional version of a hospital call light. When I'd wake up shivering and throwing up in the middle of the night, I clanked the lids. She'd run down the hall (like a highly charged Shirley MacLaine in *Terms of Endearment*) and throw her body over mine.

"You need a blanket of love!" she'd exclaim, as if *that* were a standard nurse procedure.

Her caretaker role was an emotionally exhausting job, and caretakers need advocates of their own. I asked Mom about her supporters besides my dad and her sister, Lucy. She told me about her best friend, Margy, who'd called every day after my diagnosis through my descent into kidney failure.

Mom also told me about the afternoon her friend Janet scooped her up and treated her to lunch. Taking in Mom's weary face and the visible toll from what my mom had referred to as "war," Janet said, "Liz, I'm worried about you." Mom dissolved into a heap of tears, and Janet held her tight.

Words from my dad's good college buddy Paul (who'd popped over to my parents' home one Saturday afternoon for a beer) had empowered her the most. "I'm not sure if I can handle any more," she'd told him. The marathon just seemed too long to bear.

"Look at how much you've handled already," he'd said, and that filled her up. He'd made her realize she'd already drilled the well and tapped into a deep reserve of strength. She had to trust that she'd continue to draw from that well.

The best thing Mom and I had going for us, we agreed, was our mutual ability to fall into a random belly laugh. We created our version of Where's Waldo, where we'd find the funny in the most dreadful of places. True to style, when we'd discussed her kidney donation, she'd quipped, "Come on. A couple of surgeries? It'll be a riot!"

Mom's birth name was Mildred Elizabeth, but she didn't love the name Mildred. So she went by Elizabeth and Liz for most of her life. Before surgery, she said, "I've got a name for the new kid." (She referred to the kidney as the "kid.") "How about Milly?" Mom was gifting me an original part of herself, so Milly it was.

Back on July 11, 2002, in a sterile, well-lit operating room, a surgeon had removed my mom's kidney. In an operating room nearby, another surgeon had placed it inside me. We'd traveled a long way from cinnamon toast and 7-UP.

When I'd woken, the first question I'd asked was, "Is my mom okay?"

"She's doing well," the nurse had said. "She's asking about you too. You both came through with flying colors." Relieved, I had faded back into a sleepy chemical haze.

Later, Dirk and Liza had wheeled me to Mom's room on the floor above mine. Antiseptic fumes wafted up from the vinyl floor. I remember Mom had looked tired and war-weary. Her morphine-dosed words slurred together. She'd tried to form her winning smile, but painkillers blunted the effort. Half-baked, her eyelids fluttered to stay open.

Within her slight frame in that hospital bed, I'd seen a giant of grace and goodness. I'd wanted to throw myself on top of her and be *her* blanket of love, though it would have been too painful for us both. Instead, I'd asked the nurse to inquire about reducing the morphine dosage to help with Mom's slurring. At that moment, I'd felt certain about two things—I could never repay her for all her gifts, and we'd always take care of each other.

"Thanks for asking about that," she had muttered softly, and her lips curled into a gentle smile.

"Everyone needs an Avocado, Mom," I'd said, and gently squeezed her hand.

In the seven-plus years that followed our surgeries, for every good creatinine lab result, Mom had exclaimed, "Yes!" (with a bent arm pull to signify victory). But the summer of 2002 quickly transitioned into the winter of 2009. Celebratory champagne flowed freely to honor my parents' anniversary. As the party's ample cheer lifted us up, I also tried to grasp that my mom's amazing gift was losing its life-sustaining powers. That brought me down.

Some good things last. And some good things don't.

———

PART FIVE

UNFAILING

"To love and be loved.
That is the meaning of life."

—Cheryl Strayed

66

Duped?

AFTER THE PARTY, MY EVERYDAY MOVEMENTS UNFOLDED in slow motion—my legs and ankles were taut from swelling, and my brain processed through a layer of sludge. That gradual progression was at work, like the erosion of water on stone, imperceptible from day to day, and then suddenly, the shape of the rock had changed. My labs reflected minimal remaining kidney function.

That's the remarkable thing about kidney failure; the decrease persists like a low vibration until it trembles. I'm not surprised kidney disease is known as the silent killer. Symptoms rarely occur until an advanced stage.

Soon, Milly's run would be over.

Losing kidneys. This was my pattern. I expected it. So there wasn't the same level of drama as with the original onset of kidney failure at the age of twenty-two. But after living a normal-ish life for eight years of transplant "vacation," the transition back to dialysis always feels like a robbery.

"How was your weekend, mademoiselle?" A typical greeting from Dr. Davin, the effervescent nephrologist in charge of my care. He peppered his conversations with French and started each visit with chatty tidbits. He's a delightful doctor version of your favorite uncle who consistently cracks you up at a ho-hum party.

I relished our convivial banter before we dove into kidney business, but on this day, I jumped right to what was top of mind. "I'm not ready yet." I wanted to wait until the very last minute to start dialysis because this was Milly, my mom's kidney gift, that we were talking about. Milly would be good to the last drop—and represented more than just my kidney function.

"I'd like to go on a short vacation in early February," I explained. "My labs need to hold up for the trip." I heard myself making this proclamation as if saying it out loud would make it so. I'd planned to go to Mexico for five days with my girl-friends—Rae, Carrie, Amy, Suzanne, and Liz. Half of us lived in different parts of the country and hankered for a chance to catch up on our lives. So I'd bought a ticket as if to tell the universe this *would* happen.

"We'll see. I need to track your numbers weekly," Dr. Davin said, lowering his head as he studied my file.

One week passed, and my labs inched toward the cutoff danger zone. But I remained stubbornly optimistic. Another week later, I returned to Dr. Davin's office. "How are you feeling?" He studied my face and checked my ankles by pressing his thumb over the bone.

"I'm okay?" I said unconvincingly, in the form of a question. He gripped my lab reports in his hand.

"I'm afraid it would be dangerous for you to travel with such minimal kidney function." Absent his typically jovial tone, concern saturated his words. I knew he was right; an annoying metallic taste permeated my mouth—the classic sign of kidney failure.

The airline refunded my plane ticket. My friends flew toward the sun, and I stayed behind and started dialysis. Over Skype, I got a tour of the vacation house and the love and support of my tribe. When we hung up, I fought intense fury at being separated from a normal life again. The idea that I'd be in danger without medical intervention was oppressive. I pinned my rage on the bummer that I wouldn't join them, but a canceled vacation was secondary. The real issue? The ugly force of my terrorist pinned me down again with relentless uncertainty.

In the middle of February 2010, dialysis began for the third time.

Go in. Sit down. Smile. I can handle it. Don't worry about it now. Feel it later. Emotional procrastination. Stay cheerful. See the needles. Look away. Think of something else. Nothing lasts forever. Just a poke or two.

The technician asks, "Doing okay?"

I reply, "Fine. Fine."

The technician says, "Sorry. Going to poke you again."

I think, *Just do it, damn it.* But I say, "Okay."

"Got it in," he says.

I think, *Good for you. Do you want an award for doing your awful job of driving metal needles into my skin?* But I say, "Oh, great!" Pretend smile. Polite laugh.

Was all my carefully cultivated can-do positivity a sham? Had I created this denial-fueled Pollyanna approach to live in a false reality? Had I duped myself into believing things were okay —when, in fact, they were *not* okay? Could I continue to soldier on as a be-happy-have-hope warrior, or would this stubborn illness swallow me?

Pondering these thoughts without fighting back, I wallowed. My anger erupted at how unfair and distressing and limiting it is to be held hostage by autoimmune factors that circulate in my blood and threaten to take away the healthy life I crave.

Feelings of devastation ran wildly around my brain. When I

fought to keep them out, they gained strength and muscled back in. So I exercised them to wear them out, like a pack of dogs.

People die from kidney disease. I know this all too well because a few years after I'd had lunch with Robert (the CEO that shared my FSGS diagnosis), I asked Tommy how he was doing. Tears pooled in her eyes. She said he couldn't accept living a life on dialysis. Robert had become depressed, stopped going to treatments, and died. He left his wife and young children behind. Tommy's tears spilled over the edge of her lower lashes and trickled down her face.

My mouth dropped open, and I fought the urge to burst into tears. A deep part of me connected to what Robert did, and it terrified me. Sometimes the chasm seemed so deep, and the fear so immense, that I did everything I could to avoid looking down into that vast hole. Instead, I looked up. I looked all around. Is the sky blue? Did Mom make me laugh? Did I hear a great song? Does my dog look adorable? I need to look at these things, not as a form of creative denial, or denial at all, but to see something besides that black hole.

When I'd talked to Robert about kidney disease over lunch, I'd considered him to be like me. We shared the same illness. I wish he'd have focused on some flickering light, as opposed to the darkness. Yet his despair was real, and it took the upper hand. He died from kidney disease, and the overwhelming absence of hope.

So, no. No!

My attitude is *not* a denial-fed false reality. My spring of hope is every bit as real as was his despair—it's my lifeline. I cling to it to stay afloat—for me, and for all the people in my life. So my "Pollyanna" perspective is far from naive; it's an instinct, a gift, and a choice—born of survival and incurable optimism.

Stubborn illness cannot be the winner of this emotional

wrestling match. I need to keep supporting the underdog, the one that deserves to triumph—so I cheer for the victory of stubborn hope.

67.

Adjust

RING THE BELL. DIALYSIS, ROUND THREE. DING, DING, ding. Dr. Davin suggested I learn to do treatments at home. I hesitated. In my previous dialysis experiences, showing up at an in-center clinic three times a week had helped me compartmentalize. My kidney failure life was separate from my "real" life. Did I want to position my medical treatments smack-dab in the center of my house?

Studies showed patients had better outcomes with home dialysis (more consistent lab values, fewer hospitalizations, lower mortality), so I agreed to try it. Training began. Five days a week for four weeks at a DaVita home training clinic, Dirk and I learned to operate an artificial kidney machine while my treatments took place.

Lisa, a peppy nurse, and Mark, a laid-back technician, taught us to set up the machine, manage the inventory, and order supplies. There were big bags of dialysate to make, water treatment packs to replace, and a boatload of alarm codes to learn. Lisa cheerfully gave Dirk hearty fist bumps after he'd mastered a new skill.

The last step: I received training to insert hefty-sized needles into my fistula to enable the machine to access and filter my blood. It was daunting, to put it mildly.

Four weeks later, we "graduated."

Time to get the show on the road at home, and I thought I

knew what to expect. I imagined after a day at the office I'd relax in a chair at night for a few hours, watch a show, and clean my blood. *I got this!* (You'd think by this point I'd have learned that my "plans" are a surefire way to elicit fits of laughter from God.)

When a chipper delivery guy plopped a mountain of medical supply boxes in our laundry room, I felt utterly besieged. Another fellow wheeled the seventy-five-pound machine into our bedroom, and to my dismay, it didn't compliment the decor. I'd love to report that I took it in stride, but when my medical predicament trespassed into my home, any semblance of calm was hijacked by high-strung hysterics.

Utterly overwhelmed by my life-sustaining new job, I bit Dirk's head off repeatedly for no apparent reason, to which he said, "Who are you, and what have you done with Jennifer?" I understood what he meant. I could see the tightly wound bird's-eye view of me, but I didn't know how to unspool myself.

Time, as always, helped. Eventually, I took pride in my newly acquired, self-administered nursing skills. Soon enough, the machine didn't intimidate me anymore. Training and experience transported me into the mode of a seasoned pilot—taking full command of sophisticated controls, warning lights, and cautionary alarms. Fancy that. After a rocky start, I got the hang of it.

Again, I accepted the adjustments with food and fluid limitations. Liza assisted my fluid management by giving me a collection of shot glasses to measure my ounces. The Barefoot Contessa joined me while I spent hours dialyzing in my bedroom. I absorbed plenty of other Food Network shows, learned a load of new recipes, and coveted the kitchen of Giada De Laurentiis. "It's a bummer you're on dialysis, Mom," Liza said at the dinner table one evening as she eyed her plate. "But I've got to say, it's done a lot for our family meals."

68

Thirst

STEVE CONTINUED TO CALL WITH RELATIONSHIP REPORTS. Before we could say "hola," Steve and Merly were engaged. The marriage festivities were about to unfold in Cartagena in early July. That meant I had to figure out how to receive dialysis treatments in an unfamiliar country.

A tad of terror lodged in my gut. When I thought of Colombia, I entertained images of Pablo Escobar, cocaine cartels, and violent murders in the streets. But Pablo had faced his demise in 1993.

The 2010s were upon us, ushering in the Apple iPad, East Coast storms coined "Snowmageddon" by President Obama, and relatively safe travel to Colombia.

Even so, without speaking a lick of Spanish, I couldn't imagine how a dialysis session would go. Dirk ruled the idea out of the question. But this was my brother's wedding, and I insisted on attending the celebration. Dialysis would not deter me.

So I talked to Dr. Davin about my options. He knew a nephrologist from Cartagena and provided the name of a nearby hospital. After a lengthy discussion and ample angst, I decided to go for the long weekend and skip two dialysis treatments. Dr. Davin implored me to exercise extreme caution with my food and fluids to avoid a crisis from the buildup of toxins.

Liza flew to Colombia a day ahead of Dirk and me, accompanied by my parents. Dirk and I arrived the next day without a problem and taxied to the quaint place Steve had reserved for the family. As we traveled a narrow road to the boutique hotel, the city's bright contrast of colors wowed me. Red clay roof shingles capped bright-gold-and-terra-cotta stucco buildings. A few stray dogs ambled by as the sun beamed with intense heat.

On the first evening, we boarded a large yacht with fifty guests. This is where I met and instantly loved Merly. Her personality was as colorful as the city she'd lived in all thirty years of her life. And although she was several years younger than my brother, their pairing seemed right. She worked as a lawyer in her country and matched Steve's intelligence, plus she loved movies as much as he did and analyzed plots and screenplays with the same vigor.

The boat sailed slowly into the night water, and the guests relished an abundance of food, ice-clinking drinks, and festive dancing. I restrained myself from eating and drinking. With three more days ahead without dialysis, consuming food and fluid felt dangerous. An elevated potassium level would interfere with my heart's rhythm. And fluid overload scared me too. But the festive dancing, you ask? I gave that my all.

The next day, we walked on cobbled streets through the historic Old Town, took in the palm-treed plaza, and experienced Cartagena's walled city. The sun pressed on our skin like a weighted blanket. Soon, our faces dripped with sweat. That evening, we took a dip in our shared pool and dressed for the wedding. Day two, and I had carefully controlled everything I put in my mouth to avoid problems.

Our group taxied to an old mansion in the city, a beautiful stone-walled venue. We gathered with the other guests in a cavernous interior room. I couldn't resist the mai tai offered before we sat in our designated chairs. The wedding began, and the pastor passionately performed the ceremony in rapid-fire Spanish while a translator provided the English version with a heavy accent.

Then a young man and woman performed a song. Their beautiful voices unified in a slow, even melody. The Colombian guests joined in, their voices amplified, and the song swelled. The people all around us swayed with closed eyes while the growing volume of the song swallowed us whole. After the ceremony, Steve joked, "I'm not sure . . . but I think I just joined a cult."

When the ceremony ended, out came the bubbles—shiny, iridescent soap globes floated around us. We headed downstairs to the outdoor dining and dancing reception area. I'd eaten little in the last two days, and the mai tai flared my appetite. The buffet beckoned. Along with my desire to inhale all the food, my anxiety spiked like a swift fever.

Watch it. Don't eat. Deadly heart rhythms from high potassium will surely put a damper on this glorious wedding. Dirk and I walked up to see the spread. He was hungry too and filled his plate to the brim.

"What can you eat?" he asked with concern, comparing our plates.

"I'll have some ceviche and salad. I'm okay." But the potassium-laden guacamole was right there, enticing me. "And maybe just a little guacamole," I said with fretful resignation. *Just a smidge?*

Late into the night, fireworks lit the corners of the dance floor. Costumed dancers swooped in with colorful masks during the part of the Colombian wedding celebration called *Hora Loca* (Crazy Hour). Did I mention the release of live butterflies? Festivity and a carnival-like spirit charged the atmosphere, and our family circled the dance floor with elation.

The heat remained thick late into the night. Motivated by

intense thirst, I filled a glass to the top with ice cubes. My brain taunted me with images of food and beverage fantasies like relentless spam. *Eat! Drink!* And I fought the temptations to do just that.

The next day, we boarded a bus bound for a Caribbean coastal home, the location of the after-wedding party. With broken air-conditioning, the bus became a furnace on wheels. Sweat flowed from my pores like the satirical scene in *Airplane,* where buckets of water pour from the pilot's face. Trapped in the heat without escape, and unable to drink water with abandon, agitation rocked me in my seat. I moved my tongue around my mouth to generate saliva as my empty stomach rumbled like a sputtering engine.

Worrisome thoughts played on a loop in my mind. *It's day three. What are my blood levels? Is my potassium high? Can I hold back on food and fluid for the rest of the day?*

At the oceanfront home, I grabbed a beer and gulped it in a quick second. I don't even like beer. But to this day, that beer was the most satisfying cold beverage I've ever had in my life.

Four months later, I'd see James Franco in the movie *127 Hours* play a trapped mountaineer stuck in a crevice by a boulder. Desperate for water, he drinks his urine. When he frees himself by amputating his arm, he drinks rainwater in a mad frenzy. And when a family rescues him, he chugs fresh water in a victorious, moving scene of survival.

I couldn't relate to the arm amputation, but I cried a torrent of tears when James Franco finally filled himself with unrestricted hydration at the end.

After the chilled beer went down the hatch, I berated myself. *How much fluid was that? Don't eat. Don't drink. Tomorrow is day four. Make it through today, and then you'll be home. Then you'll be safe.*

"How are you doing, Jenny?" Steve asked as we stood outside on a patio and looked at the ocean. "You seem a little tense." He must have noticed my bunched-up eyebrows as I concentrated on what not to eat. But this was his big weekend. So I tried to tuck my anxiety away.

"I did pretty well, right?" he said, and nodded toward Merly. She was chatting exuberantly with guests by the pool.

"You did great, bro."

Late the next evening, Dirk and I arrived home. I was eager to start my treatment, but it was almost midnight. After sunrise, I stepped on the bathroom scale. The prolific heat-induced sweat was helpful—I had not become overloaded with fluid despite the stretch of four days.

Hours later, after my dialysis was complete, I sealed my blood tubes in the biomedical Styrofoam box and sent them to the lab as instructed. When the results came back, my potassium was not dangerously high, despite the seductive guacamole.

I surged with relief. After traveling to another continent, swaying to Colombian music, popping bubbles, and witnessing masked Colombian "crazy hour" dancers, we were okay.

For now.

69

The Prize

AFTER THE WEDDING, WHEN SUMMER GAVE WAY TO fall, I picked up thirteen-year-old Liza after school. We headed to the pharmacy, a frequent errand, which may have sparked her conversation. "It's hard sometimes," she said, fidgeting with her backpack.

"What is?" I felt my protective-mom mode flare. Was there a bully at school? Was a teacher out of line?

"The kidney stuff—I mean . . . don't take this the wrong way," she said. Avoiding eye contact, she looked straight ahead at the road.

I pulled in a grounding breath. "It's okay, Lize. What are you thinking about?" I stole a glance at her and then turned back to face forward.

"Well, I think you do a great job. I just hope . . . I just hope it doesn't happen to me." Her hands rested on her legs, and her eyes rested on her hands.

"Oh my gosh—no!" I exclaimed. "This will not happen to you. The doctors told me this condition is not genetic," I said firmly. "It's okay for me," I continued, "but it would never be okay for you." I wanted the conviction of my words to banish her thought forever.

Relieved, she looked at me as though I'd wiped away her doubts. "I think you have an amazing attitude, Mom. You handle everything really well."

"Thanks, Lize, I try," I replied, turning briefly to take her in. My eyes on the road, I continued, "I guess through it all, I've become determined to make it the best I can."

She nodded, and I felt connected to her in a way that filled me. Gratitude flooded me as I took in the bird's-eye view of us, a mother and daughter running errands after school. There was so much more I wanted to say to her about how lucky we are and what a miracle it is to travel through this life together.

I wanted to tell her that the challenges I've endured scooped a piece out of me, but the hole has filled with a fierce appreciation for being here. For her. For Dirk. For my parents and family and friends. For robust coffee and crisp sheets and ripe avocados and spring blooms and blue skies and inside jokes, and the wonder of it all. Instead, I just rested my hand on hers and smiled.

She continued, "All I know is, I'm glad you're determined because it seems to be working. Keep doing what you're doing." I inhaled a thankful breath that Liza held a positive outlook about my health.

Soon after, I remembered the mother and daughter I'd encountered long ago at the dialysis support group. I'd traveled a long way since I'd sat in that circle with my mom. I remembered the hollow expression on that woman's face and the invisible weight that pressed her daughter into her chair.

Now Liza was a teenager, and I was in my forties. I'd guess that woman had been in her forties back when I was in my twenties. I hadn't allowed myself to empathize with her then because I'd feared her fate was my future. If only I could time travel back to that moment as my current wiser self and offer understanding and support. I wanted to return to that room and hug her and her daughter.

Through the years, my proclivity to make everything okay had garnered more depth. As life played on through my twenties, thirties, and forties, I'd learned that we will always toggle between joy and sorrow. And life is a teacher that never retires.

Decades earlier, I thought I'd crossed an imaginary line. On the other side, healthy people with perfect lives walked and biked around the lakes. They seemed so far beyond the glass barrier of my car window. That was when my brain flogged me with the question, "Why me?"

But there's no line between those who suffer and those who don't. "Why me?" is a pointless question. Suffering is inescapable—it's an unavoidable aspect of being human. There's no good answer. I realized the better question was, "Why *not* me?" and released the barrage of "whys." I'd moved forward with hard-won lessons that life is short and precious.

As Liza and I connected in the car, I fortified my determination to boost my mind-body wellness with positive imagery. Everything I could do to manifest the future I wanted for my family, I would do. We had to be okay. I had thought the stakes of this game came down to heal or fail, and healing was the prize.

But no. Maybe the real prize is living. Despite my failed kidneys and transplants, if I was still here, I didn't fail. Maybe it's quite the opposite—since I was alive, I was unfailing.

70.

Hero

A FEW WEEKS LATER, ON A SEPTEMBER SATURDAY IN 2010, Dirk and I drove an hour east to Stillwater, a charming city on the St. Croix River. We strolled through this picturesque town and enjoyed a lovely meal. After we browsed quaint shops and antique stores, we stumbled upon a sign in front of a teeny place that read "Palm and Tarot Card Reader."

"Want to?" Dirk asked as we approached.

I sat down with an eccentric woman draped with scarves and jewelry . . . right out of central casting for her role. Apparently, my palm revealed a long lifeline. She "saw" I was having struggles in 2010 but emphasized my situation would get better; 2011 promised significant improvement. I bought her story. Why not? For good measure, I changed my password to transplant2011, and prepared to remain impatiently patient.

Fifteen family members and friends had volunteered to be tested as donors since I'd started dialysis in February, including Joan, a vibrant therapist who worked at Dirk's clinic. Joan radiated life and showed up for every moment with humor, energy, and authenticity.

When Joan and fourteen other potential donors were deemed incompatible, it felt like a gut punch. But these lovely people blessed me with a bottomless cup of generosity. They offered me a gift that is mighty hard to receive—people *want* to help, and it's okay . . . let them love you.

This includes my eighty-year-old mother-in-law, who wanted to donate her kidney. Her offer, although unfeasible, felt wonderfully heartwarming. She most definitely acted on the promise she'd shared with Dirk years earlier: "I will love her." And I'd come a long way to differentiate pity from kindness.

As home dialysis continued, I struggled with anemia and its noticeable side effect, formidable exhaustion. When my hemoglobin dropped to a dangerous level, I required a blood transfusion. On the way home from this blood-boosting errand with Mom, Dirk's name flashed on my cell phone.

"I called the university today and talked to Cathy Garvey," he said. (Cathy Garvey directed the transplantation program at the University of Minnesota, and we'd known her throughout the years.) "I've set an appointment to see if I can be your donor. March seventeenth."

Dr. Davin had encouraged us to wait a year before we pursued another transplant, to allow my body a break from immune-suppressing medications. Dirk clocked that year and then pounced into action. Oh, Dirk. What are the right words when your husband tries to give you his kidney? I don't recall what I said, but I know what came to mind: *My hero.*

I turned toward Mom in the driver's seat. "Dirk talked to Cathy Garvey. He wants to get tested." I attempted a smile, but a wave of vulnerability washed over me. The enormity hit. I wanted to dissolve into a puddle of tears.

"Everyone needs a Dirk," Mom said. A compassionate smile softened her face.

That night I inhaled a book about a woman's breast cancer journey through the middle place of her life. I tucked into the corner of our striped family room sofa as the fireplace warmed the room with dancing flames. My feet shared the upholstered ottoman with Dirk's feet, sock to sock, as he relaxed in the chair beside me and answered emails. A typical evening. We sat together, sharing space, sharing our routine, sharing our lives.

The absorbing story transported me out of my life and into the author's. *I can't believe what she's been through*, came to mind. I put the book down. *How does she do it?* I looked at Dirk and recalled the activities of the day.

My mom, my third donor, accompanied me to a blood transfusion, while my husband matter-of-factly offered to give up his kidney for my fourth transplant. I chuckled at the realization. Craziness comes and goes, and we plow forward. Just another day.

Soon after Dirk's offer to donate, we felt devastated to learn Joan received a breast cancer diagnosis. It seemed wrong that illness could mess with her robustness.

Just like Tom's sudden absence from the Abbott dialysis unit in the late 1980s, the ground shook beneath us when Joan "crossed the line" from wellness to illness. The curriculum never ends—there is no line. Suffering is inescapable. The reminders keep coming that life is precious and short. I know this too well. But repeatedly learning this lesson doesn't make it easier.

We met Joan and her husband, Charlie, for dinner, and shared our love and support. The restaurant buzzed with energy. I looked around at the other tables. People sipped on cocktails and gobbled fancy-looking appetizers. How could these people enjoy a regular Saturday evening when Joan had cancer? The world had tipped. Didn't they feel it too?

Joan feared jumping off the high dive into the pool of medical chaos. Swimming in that pool was my specialty. When she leaned close and placed her hand on my shoulder, the sparkle in her eyes dulled to reveal unmistakable vulnerability. Like an eager student, she asked, "How do you do it? How do you get through all this stuff?"

The book on my nightstand came to mind. My medically busy days came to mind. And I offered the only answer I knew. "You just do."

This is how it goes: Lab draws. Car line. Grocery shopping. Math homework. Sleepovers. Bladder infections. Feeding the dog. Pharmacy runs. Snowboarding outings. Dinner dates with Dirk. Netflix. School plays. Food Network. Client meetings. Mom fun. Girlfriends. Working for Dad. Skin biopsies. Dumb jokes. Liza's tennis matches. Family dinners. *Breaking Bad* binge. Messy rooms. Clean rooms. Friends have cancer. Dog grooming. Offers to receive a new kidney.

Everyday life plus medical management. *This* is chronic illness—plowing through life while continuously toggling between wellness and illness.

Soon after, Dirk jumped at the phone's ringtone and exclaimed, "I bet it's Cathy Garvey!" I sat on the edge of the sofa as he sprang from the corner chair. His eager face expanded as he answered the call. Within a minute his cheeks collapsed, and he fell back in his seat and said, "That's not the news I wanted."

He disconnected with Cathy, pounded on the rolled arm of the chair, and shouted, "Damn it!"

"Oh no," I said. My eyes filled. We sat in silence for a moment before I spoke. "I knew we wouldn't match." Resignation wove through my words. "If fifteen people weren't a match, I didn't expect you'd be one either." I didn't want to get my hopes up after all the previous mismatches, but that was impossible. My heart dropped too.

I tried to refocus.

Visualize a transplant. See it in your mind. Appreciate your lucky list.

But fears and frustrations ricocheted inside my head.

Refocus. Refocus. Day by day. Here and now. How do you get through it? You just do. Just do. Just do. Just do it. My life is not a Nike commercial! Refocus. Refocus.

"Not me too. I was the one who was supposed to match," Dirk said, once again pounding his fist on the arm of the chair. Another strikeout. Even fourteen-year-old Liza had placed a secret call to the University of Minnesota transplant clinic to see if she could be my donor. Frustrated, she told me Cathy said she was too young to be considered. Of course she was. Bless her sweet soul.

I moved over and wrapped my arms around Dirk. "Thanks for trying, dude."

"I'm not giving up," he said. "There's got to be a way."

I replayed his convictions. *Don't give up. There's got to be a way.*

71.

Pairs

AFTER ALL THESE YEARS, I KNEW THE ROUTINE OF THIS
disease and harnessed the coping skills to endure each stage.
Kidney failure. Dialysis. Transplant. Live happy. Rinse. Repeat.
That's why it threw me when Mary, my transplant coordinator,
shared paralyzing news. She explained that my recent blood
transfusion coupled with my previous transplants and pregnancy
had elevated my antibodies.

"What does that mean?" I asked, afraid of the solemn,
steady delivery of her information.

"High antibodies reduce your ability to find a match for
another transplant," she explained.

This presented a never-before-considered possibility—what
if I couldn't get a kidney? At forty-six, a new set of fears inundated
me. What if dialysis wasn't a temporary state? Would I be on
dialysis for the rest of my life? What kind of life would that be?
I'd powered through dialysis before, and like the little engine
that could (and my U-Haul climb with Lisa toward our Queen
Anne apartment), I'd chugged my way up steep hills. But I always
got to the top. What would it take to power up a hill with a never-
ending incline?

I remembered Olga from my first dialysis experience. In her
eighties and ineligible for a transplant, I knew Olga would sit in
that treatment chair three times a week, for three to four hours
each time, until her death. But I'd never thought about that for

myself. Transplants always offered a reprieve. Kidneys equaled hope.

Keep going. I told myself this to counter the fear. *Stay here. Stay alive.*

Joan championed the get-through-it concept of *You just do.* She bolstered herself to fight like hell and maintained her sunny side. She absorbed and emitted loads of love as she powered through cancer treatment. At the time, it was beyond my grasp to ever imagine we'd lose her five years later.

You just do, until you don't. That's the terrifying reality.

Life is fragile. And sometimes, despite the fiercest determination to live, people leave us too soon.

Spring bordered summer, and Dirk, resolute as ever, pursued the paired exchange program. This is essentially a kidney exchange—people like us with a willing but incompatible donor swap with others in the same situation. If Dirk matched a person in need, then I could receive a kidney from another compatible donor. Paired exchanges bridge the gap—a tremendous breakthrough for us specifically, and for transplantation in general.

The transplant clinic required several lab tests and evaluations to determine if Dirk was healthy enough to have surgery—similar criteria to what my mom had experienced almost nine years earlier. A team of doctors at the University of Minnesota deemed Dirk a suitable candidate. He aced the tests and lifted my sense of dread; this paired exchange program would expand my slim odds. Together, we shared a helium-like lightness.

I still had high antibody levels, so finding a match remained difficult. We didn't know when (and if) anything would happen. Even so, Dirk jump-started our hope. When I hear of people shaving their heads in solidarity with loved ones who lose their hair to cancer treatment, the gesture amazes me. But hair grows back. Dirk's selfless action draped me in love and epitomized all his years of *I'm-in-this-too*.

72

Bounced

I VISUALIZED ABUNDANCE AND REMINDED MYSELF I wasn't in control.

Deep breaths.

Let go.

Just be.

In July 2011, I received a call from Mary. "Jennifer, you're due for a mammogram and Pap smear, and you should take care of it right away. I need your file up-to-date," she explained.

"You mean, *right away,* right away?" I asked. I didn't know why this had suddenly become a top priority.

"When a kidney becomes available, it happens quickly, so you shouldn't wait," she said. I immediately set up my appointments to knock these things off my list. Mary's insistence made me wonder if there was something brewing.

A week later, Mary called again. "There's a potential donor for you," she said.

"Oh my gosh." A spark ignited through my body.

"I'm not sure this will work out, Jennifer, but there's someone who may be a match." The spark intensified. "The team is looking into the compatibility."

"Well, that's super promising!"

"It's a really good kidney." In Mary's voice, I heard tempered excitement.

What if this is it? Adrenaline rushed through me. I told

my inner circle . . . and asked that they keep it on the down-low. I didn't want to jinx this with over-enthusism. Despite that, I encouraged powerful prayers and good thoughts.

Margaret, Mary's coworker, called Dirk and told him if this possibility worked for me, they'd schedule his donation surgery. So we waited to hear more news and hoped and prayed and visualized and did everything in our power to will it to be true. I wanted to be okay with everything as it was, to just be. I tried to sway my thoughts with mindfulness mantras: *Everything will be okay when you are okay with everything.* But I wanted this transplant. Was I wrong to pin my hopes on something outside of myself? It was impossible not to.

Liza, straddling eighth and ninth grade, enrolled in a summer art class, and we were on our way. The wide-open sunroof showcased a bright blue August sky. My Bluetooth setting allowed incoming calls to cut through the music with an abrupt buzz. The song stopped. Green neon letters lit up the digital dashboard. *Transplant Clinic.* I whipped my head toward Liza. "Oh . . ." slipped out, and then I froze.

"Answer it!" she screamed.

"I'm scared," I blurted out as I hit the button to receive the call. I pulled off on a side street. "Hello?" My voice cracked with nerves.

It was Mary. "The donor is a good match, and it's looking positive," she said. *Is this happening?* "He's a young man, and he would like to schedule surgery as soon as possible. Is that okay with you?"

"Anytime. Of course!" Liza started dancing an enthusias-tic stir-the-pot move in her seat. I smiled and nodded my head as if the gesture would signify a positive affirmation to Mary, who couldn't see me, and to Liza, and to the gracious universe of good things.

Mary explained that an anonymous donor from North Dakota had volunteered altruistically, meaning he didn't direct his donation so a loved one could receive a kidney. He virtuously offered this gift out of the goodness of his heart.

"Mary, you said he's young. How old is he?" I asked.

"He's twenty-five. He's been thinking about doing this for a while."

"How *long* could a twenty-five-year-old have been thinking about it?" I said with explosive gratitude. Mary and I discussed the next steps, concluded the call, and the music played. Macy Gray's "Beauty in the World" spilled through the speakers. I joined Liza in her car dance. Together we bopped side by side in our seats and sang along with Macy's raspy voice. Our arms flailed, and our hearts burst. An impossible-to-articulate joy illuminated me.

I'll never forget that moment with Liza. Her auburn hair swayed with her movement, and her smile beamed. The world's trampoline had bounced us into the air, high into the elevated space where everything looked gloriously interconnected and magnificent. An energy connected us to everyone and everything, attached us to a bigger whole, and embroidered us into the universal good that played out a new scene in this crazy life.

Liza and I wove into each other, into this lucky moment, and shared that sometimes, everything aligns. I took it all in, and thought, *I do belong here.*

Margaret called shortly afterward and asked if I could have surgery on August 19. "Yes!" I exclaimed. She said Dirk's operation would be the same day.

Liza texted her friends. I called Mom. She was standing by to help with everything, anything, as she does. I called my friend Jane, and she offered to handle Liza's drop-offs and pickups from school. Phone calls. Emails. Texts. The word spread quickly to our friends and family, and the excitement everyone shared lifted me. Margaret changed the date to August 25 due to operating room availability.

There were many layers of goodness besides my husband's generosity; a total stranger in this world stepped up to improve my life significantly. The world brightened as if a cold winter day had instantly burst into spring.

Dirk's extra kidney and big heart offered renewal for a sixty-something diabetic man in North Dakota. Dirk's loving intentions directed toward me jump-started a double whammy of do-good.

I imagined the moment the North Dakota man received the news he had been waiting for—the call that would change his life. I considered his family and friends and their inevitable excitement for his opportunity, and I felt an amplified connection between all of us.

Dirk didn't focus on his kidney's destination; instead, he focused on our surgeries. One of us wanted to be home with Liza while the other was in the hospital, so Margaret arranged Dirk's surgery for September 1, one week after mine.

Four surgeries—my altruistic donor, me, Dirk, and the man who would receive Dirk's kidney—launched into motion by Dirk and a remarkably selfless young man I'd never met.

73

Superheroes

WHAT MOTIVATES ALTRUISTIC KIDNEY DONORS TO volunteer their kidney to a person they don't know? Abigail Marsh, a psychology researcher from Georgetown University, studied the brain for answers.

After scanning brains from benevolent, altruistic donors, Marsh and the researchers discovered these folks had an 8 percent larger than average amygdala and a heightened sensitivity to other people's fear and distress. Notably, when Marsh interviewed these charitable individuals, they consistently claimed they were not special.

Oh, but they are. I'd say these people are rare gems that sparkle in this world.

Consider heroes like Brian Glennon, a stay-at-home father to four children, who executed kindness sharing on a grand level. When forty-seven-year-old Brian decided to give in a meaningful way, he donated his kidney. Altruistically. To a stranger. Just because.

Megyn Kelly interviewed him on the *Today Show* and asked why he didn't just sign up for volunteer work instead. And his answer was, "We all have two kidneys, and we only need one."

So Brian had donation surgery at Saint Barnabas Medical Center in New Jersey. His recipient was a woman named Hayley. And Brian was thrilled to free Hayley from the dialysis treatments she required to stay alive.

Brian met Hayley for the first time on the *Today Show* episode. After a warm embrace, Hayley said, "Thank you for saving my life."

Brian looked bashful and a little embarrassed, and said he wasn't sure how to respond. But like a humble superhero, he replied, "You're welcome. I'm happy your daughter will have more time with you."

When Brian donated his kidney, he never expected his gift of life would keep on giving. But boy, did it ever. Because after Brian donated to Hayley, Hayley's daughter (who wasn't a match for her mom) donated her kidney to a stranger. And that stranger had an incompatible donor who donated their kidney to a stranger. It went on and on and on. People with willing but incompatible donors could get a kidney when their loved ones matched other people in need. Brian's altruism was the first domino, and it cascaded into a forty-six-person kidney chain.

Every story begins with a domino moment that starts a chain of events.

Abigail Marsh might find Brian has a larger than average amygdala, and I'd say he's a hero. Remarkable people like Brian epitomize the best of abundance and kindness. Imagine it. He gave of himself without any considerations of politics, age, or religion. With a pure heart, he changed the world by doing more for others than he expected in return. What an inspirational example of connection by kindness.

There is beauty in the world.

Days Before the Transplant

Dr. Naim Issa, the transplant nephrologist in charge of my care, championed my case. I instantly liked him. His dark chocolate eyes and close-cut dark hair warmed his welcoming face. He took the time to know me, beyond my diagnosis, and set out to make this transplant my best. To that end, he scheduled proactive plasmapheresis before my surgery—treatments that separate my plasma from my blood to remove antibodies that could cause rejection and FSGS damage. I would do these treatments regularly for the first year after my transplant.

August 25, 2011

The day had arrived. Dirk and I pulled into Fairview University at 5:30 a.m. In my hospital room, I donned a gown and tucked into the bed. A nurse recorded my vitals. Then we waited.

Infection fears had baked into my cells ever since the rapid spread of sepsis after Liza's birth. *I'll take one kidney, please. Hold the sepsis.* This fear was at the top of Dirk's mind too. So Dr. Young, my go-to infection specialist, ordered IV antibiotics before surgery to cover and protect me.

At 1:00 p.m., I entered the pre-op prep area, and the anesthesiologist resident introduced himself. He looked like he was sixteen. His youthful appearance and timid personality wouldn't inspire my confidence if he were a babysitter, let alone a guy who administers powerful drugs.

We were all just talking like you do, filling the pre-surgery space with words. I joked with Liza, "Maybe they can do something to enhance my boobs in there too." She soaked up the comic relief.

The youngster doctor wheeled me toward the operating room. It was happening so fast. Dirk hugged me first, tight, his eyes misty. Then Liza hugged me hard. Mom and Dad leaned in and wrapped me with sentiments of good luck. As the doctor wheeled me away from them, Liza ran up and whispered in my ear, "Don't forget to ask them about that bonus boob job." Leave it to Liza, she left me with the last laugh.

I addressed the teenage-looking doctor from my position on the stretcher and said, "I want to be sure to get the antibiotic before I go under."

"I don't know anything about that," he said.

"I need the antibiotic. Please look into it. I had sepsis once; I want to be sure to get covered with an antibiotic." Blank stare. "Who can I talk to?" I begged.

"I'll check it out." Would he? Panic rushed through me. The OR was green, sterile, and icy cold. I asked the anesthesiologist again if I could get the IV antibiotics before they put me to sleep, so I'd know I'd received them.

He seemed unsure. Then, in a flash, the chief anesthesiologist swooped in. He connected a syringe to my IV. That was the last thing I remember.

I woke up in a post-operative recovery room. Groggy. Foggy. In pain. Dirk and Liza appeared, and I saw tears in their eyes. I asked if everything went okay; they didn't answer me. The nurse took my temperature. It was elevated.

I repeatedly asked the nurse if they'd given me the IV antibiotic. He didn't know. He also didn't care. It terrified me that an infection could be causing my fever. I told him about Dr. Young and my previous sepsis episode. I pleaded with him to call her. He said my blood pressure was very low and his job was to ensure the kidney received enough fluids. He worked urgently on what he thought was the first course of action required, and dread pounded with my every heartbeat.

Dirk called Dr. Young. The nurse, visibly irritated (exemplified by his short and dismissive tone), said, "Antibiotics are not my priority." He asked Dirk to move aside.

Then a doctor I didn't know came in and said I'd *not* received the antibiotics. I launched into a shaky voice explanation of Dr. Young's plan and my previous sepsis scares. He stood over me, composed and detached. As I looked up at his unfamiliar face, I dissolved with vulnerability.

After the doctor left, another nurse came in and said I *had* received the antibiotics. *Why doesn't anybody know what is going on?* Tense and frightened, I floated in and out from the anesthesia. I woke up with cloudy confusion. *How late is it? Did everyone go home? Where are my doctors?*

I learned later that when the surgeon placed the kidney, milky fluid appeared instead of urine. An infection had parked in my bladder. It became stuck, like gridlock in traffic, because nothing had been moving through my system without a functioning kidney. My surgeon's first report to Dirk and Liza sounded discouraging, because he hadn't expected the infection. He said he'd done his best. That's why Dirk and Liza cried when they first saw me. They didn't have any glowing reports to pass on.

Later, Dirk told me this experience had toppled him more than any of the other health scares he'd endured, including the sepsis episode, because they'd shut him out. No family members allowed. He'd never heard that before, and he felt sure I would die.

He paced with Liza in the hospital halls. I can picture the scene. His shoulders rounded, head down, Liza's eyes wide, looking to Dirk for answers but butting up against his brooding silence. I didn't know this was taking place in the halls outside my room, where I tensed with worry about the antibiotic and whether I had received it.

At 2:00 a.m., they transferred me to the ICU. Dirk and Liza walked into the room slowly. It elated me to see their faces because I thought they were asleep at home. They'd never left the hospital.

Dirk called my mom and dad and told them there were complications and they should come back. At 2:30 a.m., my parents walked into the ICU too. I considered all the time that Mom and Dad had camped out with me at this hospital, and now Liza and Dirk were here too. My people.

I received a constant infusion of IV fluids and medications. My incision hurt, so I didn't want to move. Infection fears left traces of trauma, so sleep seemed the best option to escape the anxiety. Thankfully, the infection did not run rampant. It cleared from my system compliments of antibiotics and the flushing powers of my new kidney.

In two days, I was in a much better post-operative state, and they transferred me to the sixth floor. Familiar things followed. A fresh scar. A painful walk to get moving. Medications. The absolute glee in drinking a bevy of beverages. And best of all, the indelible love of my family.

In 1938, scientists began a now-famous study to uncover clues to health and happiness. The Harvard Study of Adult Development, still ongoing, tracks the lives of participants over the trajectory of their lifetimes and compiles measures of their well-being. (The study initially included Harvard sophomores and expanded to include Boston inner-city residents and wives.) An interesting result rose to the top of their findings.

Initially, many participants claimed they desired future money or fame to achieve happiness. Over time, guess what emerged as the most important measure of happiness from the participants? Close relationships. This study reveals steady relationships have the power to delay physical and mental decline over a lifespan.

I love this study. It dispels the quick-fix notion that an elusive key to happiness opens a door into a technicolor happy land. Not so. Over time, steady investments in relationships pay off with happier, healthier returns. I thought about my burning drive for independence when I was twenty-two years old, and my utter devastation when I lost it.

Throughout these years, I've realized that independence by itself is incomplete. I wanted to stand solidly on my own two feet, but I never wanted to stand alone on an island. Mutual dependence makes families, friendships, marriages, communities, and human kindness flourish.

Maybe I'd realized the meaningful life that I'd hoped for all along. How lovely to be braided into life with the people I love.

Liza started ninth grade during my hospital stay. It was the first year she wasn't required to wear a tartan plaid skirt and a navy polo shirt. So she texted me a fashion show of outfit possibilities for her first non-uniform week. Although I was sad to miss the first day of her high school send-off, we celebrated the reason it wasn't possible.

Four days later, I left the hospital. On my first night home with the three of us under one roof, euphoria set in from the best medicine. I felt like I'd clicked my red heels together three times and soaked in the wisdom of Dorothy. "There's no place like home."

With one surgery down and one to go, we prayed that Dirk's operation would prove less complicated.

74

Together

THE DAY BEFORE DIRK'S SURGERY, LIZA STAYED AT my parents' home, and my mom would drop her at school the next morning. That night, Dirk and I flipped and flopped restlessly in bed, punched our pillows, and stared at the clock.

"I can't sleep," I grumbled, unnecessarily. He knew.

"I can't either." Middle of the night statements of the obvious. We'd set the alarm for 4:00 a.m., but we were up before the chime sounded. At 4:45, a cab pulled into the driveway, and we walked through the darkness to get into the back seat. Too early for words, I grabbed Dirk's hand, and we rode in silence.

September 1, 2011

Everything happened quickly when we arrived at the hospital. In a bright white room, Dirk put on the familiar faded, dreary blue gown and robe. The hospital wardrobe I knew so well seemed out of place on him. Flat on a stretcher, he arranged the sheet over his legs. I covered him with a blanket and swallowed hard to push down the lump in my throat.

Anesthesiologists came in to assess him. A nurse poked his arm to place an IV in a vein. Her first attempt failed, and a bloody mess stained the sheets.

Dirk grimaced as the nurse tried again. He had been stoic and matter-of-fact about the surgery until this moment. When his eyes began to glisten with vulnerability, he squeezed them shut. The second IV attempt was successful, and that butcher lady left the room.

Another nurse bounced in to greet us and asked Dirk if he was anxious. He turned to me, his lower lip quivering, and nodded yes. I pushed the nurse out of my way and jumped on top of him. As we shed tears and hugged, I wanted to melt into him and take it all away. This was insane. He was undergoing surgery on my behalf! What were we doing here?

The nurse gave him a sedative, and the tension around his mouth eased. In seconds, he fell asleep. Two other nurses wheeled him out of the room toward the OR, and I took comfort in knowing he was in a peaceful anesthetic slumber.

The pain from my incision intensified as edginess constricted my muscles. My shoulders clenched, my abdomen compressed against my ribs, and my neck contracted. Nine years earlier, my mom's kidney donation surgery happened within hours of mine. I woke up to the instant news that she was doing well and then fell asleep from heavy sedation.

But for Dirk's surgery, I remained fully alert to worry. And wait. And worry. And wait. A hammer of guilt struck me. I had a glimpse into the intensity my parents, Dirk, and Liza had endured for all the surgeries when I'd been the one under.

Sore and slow-moving, I walked from Dirk's hospital room through a skyway to an attached clinic and checked in for the treatment Dr. Issa had ordered to protect my new kidney. While resting in a hospital bed myself over the next two hours receiving plasmapheresis, I ruminated over the mind-blowing events taking place. A week ago, I'd received a kidney from a man I didn't know. Today, Dirk's kidney was being removed on my behalf and transported to North Dakota to save another man we didn't know. We've experienced a lot of astonishing days, but this one really took the prize.

After my procedure, I gingerly paced in the waiting room. My mom joined me with her all-encompassing support. Hours passed. Finally, Dirk's surgeon, Dr. Pruett, called and said the surgery was over and had gone well. I let out a monstrous sigh and wiped the tears that spilled. Dr. Pruett said, "He'll be in recovery for two to three hours, and you can see him after that."

At three o'clock in the afternoon, a couple of fellows wheeled Dirk into room 504 on 6-D. Vaseline-textured goop oozed from his eyes. His voice sounded raspy and weak, and pain twisted his face. I reached for his arm and squeezed lightly. He appeared momentarily confused when he glanced at the IV tubing connected to a saline bag. Then his understanding sharpened, and he looked at me with a combined expression of incredulousness and accomplishment. Like the liquids dripping in his line, emotionality dripped from his face.

A wave of energy pulsed from my hand into his skin. In his wide-open eyes, I saw our shared history and became overwhelmed by our connection. The night we became engaged flashed back, when Dirk said, "We'll deal with whatever we need to deal with. Together."

That "we" had signaled hope for a future. Our future. But I could never have imagined that our "we"-ness would lead to this.

I'd wrestled the restrictive cloak of false perfection and my "damaged goods" identity alongside this man. He didn't place me on a pedestal or expect me to pump positivity when my emotions veered otherwise. A calming and essential realization washed over me: there's no shame in being an imperfect human. How lovely to display and accept our imperfections together. Isn't that the quintessence of genuine connection? Come as you are.

As I continued to squeeze Dirk's IV-free arm tenderly, a runaway tear trickled down his cheek. I wiped it away with the thumb of my other hand. A tired but robust smile spread across his face, and in a strained voice, he said, "We did it, Jen."

At the tail end of my twenty-second year, I stumbled and fell. Then I stood up and stumbled again and stood up and stumbled many more times. But every time, helping hands hoisted me back up. So this I know: where we find helpers outstretching their hands, we find hope.

I'll forever marvel at the wonder of it all. How lucky it is to be alive and connected to people I adore. I learned a long time ago that there's tremendous power in many things I can't see, but throughout all these decades, the potency of love has proven to be the strongest of all.

Epilogue

AS I WRITE THIS, THE KIDNEY MADE POSSIBLE BY Dirk and my anonymous, altruistic donor (over eleven years ago!) continues to provide a fabulous dialysis vacation. Dirk recovered beautifully and remains healthy, happy, and my hero. Liza, now in her mid-twenties, is diving headfirst into her future with ardent independence and big dreams.

Knowing I'll likely need another kidney in the future, Liza pursued testing at the Mayo Clinic to see if she can donate hers when the time comes. Far from being a fourteen-year-old, she'd just celebrated her twenty-fifth birthday. And in a fit of complicated and joyful tears, we learned we are a direct match.

My feelings about this are multilayered and enormous—I keep thinking about her precious premature hand gripping mine after she was born. How fiercely I wanted to protect her from any harm, and still do. That hand still squeezes mine, but now she wants to protect me. As we often say to each other when we process it, it's so much love.

The plasmapheresis treatments that Dr. Issa recommended (in collaboration with Dr. Riad) have improved the course of my FSGS and proteinuria. I continue to receive treatments twice a month—the likely reason this kidney has lasted longer than the others. Here's hoping it will provide many more years.

My fistula comes in handy for plasmapheresis. But aside

from medical appointments, I hide the bulging vein on my left arm with chunky bracelets. Years earlier, I'd asked my doctor if we could make my arm look better. He recommended I talk to the same surgeon who created the fistula years ago.

That surgery had been so traumatic, so I had huge reservations about seeing that country-singing jackass again. But he was the best guy to answer my questions; I made an appointment.

I presented my fistula, told him I'd had a transplant, and asked if he could reduce the prominent bulge. He said I should keep it as a useful insurance policy in case I'd need to use it again. He underscored that same refrain: transplants are a vacation from dialysis.

When I thanked him for his opinion, I reminded him he'd performed the initial surgery. (We didn't rehash his outburst when he thought he'd punctured my lung. "Goddamn nephrotics!")

Recognition lit up his face. "Oh, I remember you!" he exclaimed. "I was so worried about you. You were so young, and I didn't know what would become of you. You had such fragile veins and seemed so sick. Look at you now!" He seemed genuinely delighted. Although we had met decades before, I felt like he saw me for the first time.

"I know!" I agreed with his look-at-you-now observation. He was right. I'd come a long way. "I have a good life."

"Are you married?" he asked hesitantly.

"Yes!"

"Do you have any children?" he asked with wide eyes and heightened energy.

"Yes! We have a daughter." My voice became animated and rose with his energy. He marked a tough time that seemed so long ago. I was happy to tell him about my life now.

To my amusement, he smiled and pumped playfulness into his final question, "Do you have a dog?" (As if a dog would seal the deal.)

"Yes!" I beamed, and we both laughed. If only he'd asked if I had a house, he'd have been right in step with my engagement checklist.

"I'm thrilled to know you're doing so well—I don't think I'd have predicted it all those years ago. How wonderful you came to see me! You've made my day."

And he made mine. I left his office elated. That crazy guy was truly happy for me, and it erased the previous nightmare. As I walked through the sliding doors of that clinic, greeted by a bright blue sky, I wanted to shout out to the world, "It's settled. I really am so much more than a 'goddamn nephrotic!'"

Onward. I can't predict or control what's ahead, but this I know: as long as I seek beauty in the world, I will find it.

Acknowledgments &
Gratitude

It takes a village to stay alive—and it takes a village to write a book. I have so many people to thank on both counts!

To the all the dedicated transplant doctors, surgeons, providers, coordinators, SIPC nurses, lab technicians, cooks, valet parkers, greeters—all the dedicated staff and volunteers—at the University of Minnesota Medical Center, Fairview. And a special shout out to Dr. El-Rifai and my coordinator Sam. This book and my life would not be possible without you.

To Dr. Issa—Thanks for putting your brilliant brain into my case and sharing my determination to make my life the best it can be. I'm so grateful for your care and appreciate how you see me as a person, not a disease. It makes all the difference.

To the crew at M Health Apheresis—Thanks for your proficiency and expertise. Hanging out with you all for many hours over many weeks is more "fun" than one might expect. You make a medical situation not so bad—a bit like catching up with friends for coffee (except with large needles and humming machines). But still. I'm grateful for your good-natured, accomplished staff.

To all the hardworking nurses and technicians at DaVita—You make a tough situation better by doing what you do with expertise and bright smiles.

To Dr. Davin—You are one of a kind, and I am very grateful for your big brain, random bouts of French (Bonjour!), and charming nature. Plus, all the wonderful nurses at your office are amazing, caring people. We've traveled on a long journey together. Here's wishing you a relaxing and lovely retirement!

To the doctors and nurses at the neonatal intensive care unit at Hennepin County Medical Center—Your special skills are a gift to all of us who trust our fragile and precious preemies to your care.

To Dr. Brown—Thanks for showing me that doctors not only have an incredible dedication to their field but also really care about their patients.

To all the kidney patients and their families—It's a hard road, but the people we love make the ride worthwhile. Here's to your continued strength, perseverance, and life force. We're in this together.

To the National Kidney Foundation—You walk alongside kidney patients to improve our lives. Your efforts for prevention, advocacy, and reducing barriers to living donation are making a big difference. I'm so proud to be working with you on this mission.

To the team at LifeSource—You are the ones behind the scenes to educate people about organ donation, transport the organs, comfort families in their grief, and work at the intersection of life and death. Thank you for your important work.

To my family—Starting with my favorite husband. Dirk! I can't imagine being in this life without you. All those years ago when we got hitched, you believed in my future. And our life together has been beyond a dream come true. In my wildest dreams, I could never have envisioned just how lovely it has unfolded.

Mom! It's always a love-fueled riot. How much gratitude can I hold? Your gifts are unmeasurable, and your unconditional, even-keeled, all-in love is the kind of magic I hope to model for Liza. We are all better people because of your grace.

Dad! You're my role model for positivity. I couldn't possibly plow through any of this stuff without the tools you've provided. It'd be impossible to catalog all the life lessons you've given me, and for that, I'm so grateful.

Steve, Merly, the McInnis crew, Millers, McNultys, Bob Cramer, and Marcy Wallace—Thanks for being my people. It's lovely to belong to you all.

To Lisa, Cindy, Susan, and Gillian—I love how we've stuck together even though we live far apart. It's been fun to transition into real and responsible adults with you, although our crazy college years are ones I'll always cherish. And a warm hello to all the Pi Phis!

To Nick: I'm grateful that our recent conversation, the first in over thirty years, recapped my top life lesson—we're all just humans trying to manage uncertainty and find joy. I'm delighted you're in a good place and living a lovely life.

To the Luckies—From kindergarten and beyond, we've banded together. And we'll keep doing what we always do: listen, cry, offer tissues, soften it all with humor, laugh lightly, laugh loudly, weep, whisper, shout, and laugh again. I'm so happy we get to muddle through the thick and thin of our lives together.

To my Cherished Friends—so many of you (and you know who you are!) Life is so much more fun because all of you are in it with me.

To Kate Hopper—Oh my goodness, Kate! We've done splendid work together. Because of you, this memoir is tighter, better, and more profound. I see your advice on every page. Thank you. You guided me gently while you encouraged me to be brave and write the truth.

To Julie Burton—You have inspired me in tremendous ways! Thank you for creating spaces to write and connect and get the fires burning. The Twin Cities Writing Studio, ModernWell, and your die-hard support fueled me to keep on chugging out pages.

To Nina Badzin—My teacher, my friend. You are incredible and jazzed me up about writing with your razor-sharp insights and enthusiasm for making me better. Your expertise infuses each writing session with tips that propelled me to find the fun in this pursuit! Now that's an impressive trick.

To Herta Feely and Writer's Ally—It was you who made me truly believe this book would reach others. Herta, you coached me to finish the marathon. With your wisdom, insights, and observant cheerleading, you brought this memoir into its best and final form. I can't thank you enough, and will never forget the moment you said, "This book is highly publishable."

To Linda Sivertsen—Your encouragement. Your heart. Your stick-to-it cheerleading. Your energy. Your expertise. It all adds up to big magic. Thank you, friend! You gave me the boost of wind that helped me fly.

To Brooke Warner, Lauren Wise, and the team at She Writes Press—Thank you for the green light! Thank you for believing that this story is worth sharing broadly. And thank you for helping me every step of the way to make it a reality!

To Caitlin Hamilton Summie—From our first conversation, our first three minutes, really, I knew we'd make a great team. Thank you for your publicity magic!

To the Thursday girls—We are doing incredible things together! Each one of you offers so much wisdom, craft, humor, and heart. You are empowering, wise, and inspirational women! And your support lifts me way, way up. Carolyn once said during one of my kidney setbacks, "We got this!" I'm still smiling over that simple statement of our bond and unity.

* To my Liza!—How could I not end with you? My miracle. My favorite human. Even though you're now a brave, hilarious, loyal, independent woman, the powerful grip we share will connect us always. 150 percent. Trust me on this, keep shining your unique light and you will illuminate the world.

Facts and Resources

Chronic Kidney Disease (CKD) Facts

- An estimated 37 million American adults have CKD.
- Millions more are at increased risk.
- The two main causes of CKD are diabetes and high blood pressure.
- CKD causes high blood pressure, and high blood pressure causes CKD.
- Protein in the urine means CKD is present.
- African Americans and Black individuals have an increased risk of CKD.
- Pacific Islanders have an increased risk of CKD.
- American Indians have an increased risk of CKD.
- Seniors (over sixty) have an increased risk of CKD.
- A family history of kidney failure also puts you at high risk for CKD.

Early Detection Is Critical

Early detection can help prevent the progression of kidney disease and kidney failure. Simple tests can detect CKD: 1) blood pressure, 2) urine albumin (protein), and 3) serum creatinine.

Kidney Transplant and Waiting List Facts

- About 100,000 Americans are on the waiting list for a kidney.
- Only 25,000 people receive a kidney transplant each year.

- ○ Every day, seventeen people die while waiting on the list.
- ○ Donation gives people a chance. Donation saves lives.

Do you need a kidney or want to learn more about becoming a donor? Please visit the National Kidney Foundation website (**www.kidney.org**) for comprehensive information and resources. The National Kidney Foundation is the source of the above information and statistics.

THE POWER OF YES SAVES LIVES!

Will you consider signing up to be a donor today?

1. You can find comprehensive information from the Donate Life website at **donatelife.net**. Learn all about it and get all your questions answered. Then if you choose, click on **Register to Be a Donor**. Registration takes less than a minute. It's a small investment of time for such a huge gesture.

2. You can also sign up at your local **Department of Motor Vehicles** or go to **organdonor.gov**. This site will also take you to a registration form. Fill it out, hit send, and feel proud—you have just done something so meaningful. Because here's the thing, Donate Life reports that although 95 percent of Americans are in favor of being a donor, only 56 percent are registered. Let's narrow that gap and save many lives through the power of yes.

3. Spread the word. Tell your family and friends so they can support and gain inspiration from your decision.

Kindness is love in action. And the kind actions of donors live on by sharing the gift of life, of time, and the luxury of memory-making for so many. As just one voice in the transplant community, I am so grateful for the power of yes. So if you feel it is right for you, please consider helping many others like me.

Thank you!

Credits

The author is grateful for permission to reprint:

Quotation from *The Book of Bebb*, 2001 Paperback Edition (HarperCollins Publishers), Source ISBN: 978-0-06-251769-2, Source Chapter Open Heart, Chapter 17, Page Range 251, reprinted by permission of the Frederick Buechner Literary Assets, LLC.

Quotation from A. Joseph Campbell Companion, *Reflections on the Art of Living by Joseph Campbell*, 1991, reprinted by permission of the Joseph Campbell Foundation (jcf.org).

ABOUT THE AUTHOR

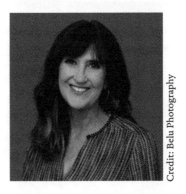

Credit: Belu Photography

JENNIFER CRAMER-MILLER is a writer, speaker, and happiness seeker. Her work is featured in the *Brevity Blog*, *The Sunlight Press*, *Grown & Flown*, *Mamalode*, *Medium*, the *Erma Bombeck Blog*, the *Kindness Blog*, the *Star Tribune*, and the *Minnesota Physician*. She is the 2023-2026 Board Chair and a contributing writer for the Minnesota National Kidney Foundation. She also works as a patient advocate (named Joy Scouter) to help others manage uncertainty to boost hope and joy. You'll find her essays on her website at www.jennifercramermiller.com.

Jennifer finds a whole lotta joy living with her funny, lover-of-golf husband and fluffy, lover-of-treats pup in a suburb of Minneapolis, Minnesota.